About Andrea McGinty

Andrea McGinty is a trailblazing entrepreneur, speaker, and dating coach who has spent over 30 years transforming the dating industry with her fresh, results-driven approaches. Known for her practical, graciously direct, and no-nonsense advice, she empowers individuals—particularly those over 50—to navigate the complexities of modern dating with confidence and clarity.

In the 1990s, Andrea launched It's Just Lunch (IJL), an iconic matchmaking service that expanded to over 110 locations worldwide and set up more than 30,000 first dates. After selling IJL to private equity, she saw that modern singles needed a roadmap to navigate the vast world of online dating.

In the 2020s, Andrea launched 33000Dates.com, a pioneering platform that combines the convenience of online dating with a strategic, personalized approach to help singles meet compatible partners. Her innovative platform now connects "Second Actors" with a much wider pool, surpassing the limits of traditional matchmaking. Andrea's insight and experience have led many over 50 to new relationships and happiness. She thrives on happy clients and loves her unique business.

©2025 by Andrea McGinty
All Rights Reserved.

No part of this book may be used or reproduced by any means: graphic, electronic, or mechanical, including photocopying, recording, taping, or by any information storage retrieval system without the written permission of the author, except in the case of brief quotations embodied in critical articles and reviews. Because of the dynamic nature of the Internet, any web addresses or links contained in this book may have changed since publication and may no longer be valid. Although every precaution has been taken to verify the accuracy of the information contained herein, the author and publisher assume no responsibility for any errors or omissions, so no liability is assumed for damages that may result from the use of the information contained within. The views expressed in this work are solely those of the author and do not necessarily reflect the views of the publisher, whereby the publisher hereby disclaims any responsibility for them.

ATTRIBUTIONS

Interior Text Font: Minion Pro
Interior Title Fonts: Minion Pro
Front Cover: Robbie Grayson III
Editor: Hollie McKay

BOOK PUBLISHING INFORMATION

Paperback ISBN: 979-8-3305-1243-0
Hardcover ISBN: 979-8-3306-7858-7

Book Industry Standards and Communications (BISAC)

1) Family & Relationships: Life Stages / Midlife
2) Family & Relationships: Love / Romance
3) Family & Relationships: Dating

33000Dates Publishing
33000Dates.com

33000 Dates
Publishing
New York • London

THE WORLD'S LEADING ONLINE DATING EXPERT SHARES **166** PRACTICAL, NO-NONSENSE, STEP-BY-STEP APPROACHES TO ROMANCE

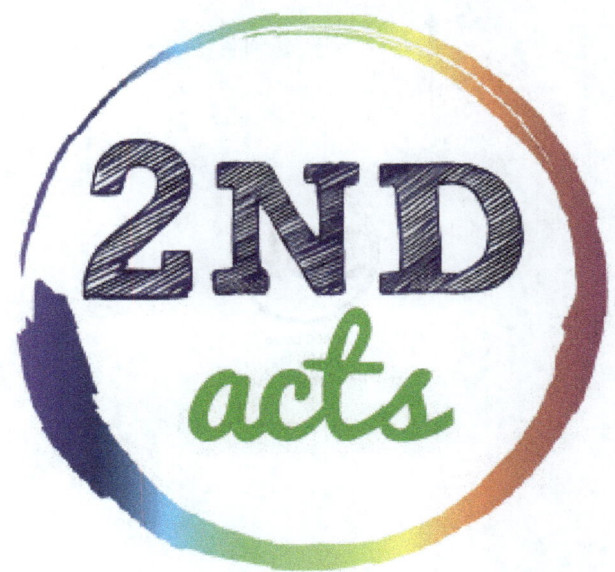

WINNING STRATEGIES FOR DATING OVER 50

ANDREA McGINTY

FOUNDER OF IT'S JUST LUNCH AND 33000DATES.COM

**33000 Dates
Publishing
New York • London**

To my dad, Jack McGinty—

Dad, how can I ever express how much you mean to me and all you've taught me? From family, love, and sports to business, a love of reading, and open-mindedness—you shaped my world. I'll never forget when I got fired from my day job while starting my first company. You said, "That's okay, honey. Many successful people get fired… and multiple times." Then, smiling, "Let's go get a pizza." You showed humility, treated everyone with respect, and were a fierce advocate for women in the workplace, instilling a solid work ethic in each of your six children. You are truly one of a kind, and I'm incredibly lucky to be your daughter. This is for you, Dad. I miss you every day.

second actor \ n

1: an individuals, typically over 50, who re-enters the dating world with newfound intention and purpose | 2: an individual who, after a "first act" shaped by marriage, widowhood, or choices made without a full grasp of their needs, now brings a wealth of life experience and a clearer sense of self to the pursuit of meaningful connection. | 3: an individual who is more self-aware of what they want and need in a romantic partner, more cognizant of optionality, and more deliberate in choice-making.

Contents

DISCLAIMER
HOW TO USE THIS BOOK | 1

chapter 1

HOW IT ALL BEGAN (1)

chapter 2

GETTING YOUR MIND RIGHT (25)

#1 Hire a Dating Expert (25)
#2 Be Sure You Are Ready… to Go All In (30)
#3 Attitude Is Everything (36)
#4 Embrace the Unique Challenges of Dating After 50 (38)
#5 Remind Yourself That There Are 3 Ways
    to Approach Dating (44)

chapter 3

BUILDING YOUR BRAND (49)

#6 Take a Business-Minded Approach (49)
#7 Put Work into Personal Branding (50)
#8 Take Time Out to Develop Your Story (53)
#9 Turning to Your Friends (54)
#10 Crafting the Dating Elevator Pitch (58)
#11 Refine the Pitch to a Catchy Tagline (59)
#12 Cue the Makeover (65)
#13 Trim (or Better Yet Shave) That Beard (66)
#14 Get Moving (67)
#15 Botox/Filler Rules and Regulations (68)
#16 Seek Out a Personal Shopper (69)
#17 Configure Your Color Scheme (70)
#18 Pay Attention to "Down There" (71)
#19 Tailor Those Clothes and Accessories (72)
#20 Mani (and Heck, Why Not the Pedi) Time (73)
#21 Whiten That Smile (74)
#22 Professional Photos Are a Must (75)
#23 Master the Art of Listening (76)
#24 The Importance of Being Well-Read (77)
#25 Have a Social Media Presence (78)
#26 Be Mindful of Those Negative Nips (79)
#27 Ditch the One-Track Type (80)
#28 Nobody Wants to Be on Dating Apps Forever (83)
#29 Commit to an All-In Effort for at Least (92)

chapter 4

NAVIGATING THE DIGITAL LANDSCAPE

#30 Diversify Your Dating Portfolio (95)
#31 Platforms to Go For (97)
#32 Platforms to Avoid (104)
#33 Some "Maybe" Platforms to Consider (108)
#34 Pay to Play (113)
#35 Engage, Engage (114)
#36 Farewell the Common Misconceptions (115)
#37 Avoid Early Blustering and Burnout (117)

chapter 5

CRAFTING THE PERFECT PROFILE

#38 Keep It Short, Sweet, and Quirky (121)
#39 Ask a Question (123)
#40 Throw in a Super Bowl Ad if You Desire (124)
#41 Target Your Niche. Know Your Niche (125)
#42 Choosing the Best Photos (126)
#43 Show, Not Tell (133)
#44 The Low-Down on Featuring Others (134)
#45 Inject Humor into Your Profile (135)
#46 The Want-Kids-Someday Prompt (140)
#47 Be Careful of Cliches (141)
#48 Putting Your Politics Out There with Caution (144)
#49 Seek Feedback from Friends (145)
#50 Update Your Profile Regularly (146)
#51 Bypass the Scammers (147)
#52 The Two-Week Travel Dating Rule (148)
#53 Looking for Tea and Red Flags? Not So Fast (150)
#54 Outside the Online Dating Sphere (151)

chapter 6

THE ART OF THE FIRST DATE

#55 Setting Expectations (163)
#56 To Call or Not to Call (164)
#57 Give a "Which" Day Works (168)
#58 Managing Nerves (169)
#59 Choosing the Right Time and Place (170)
#60 Share Your Cell (173)

#61 Prep: Stay Safe, but Don't Ruin Potential Magic (174)
#62 Dressing Appropriately (178)
#63 Be Punctual (179)
#64 The Sober Factor (180)
#65 Questions to Ask (181)
#66 Questions Not to Ask (183)
#67 More Things Your Date Doesn't Want to Hear (189)
#68 How to Handle the "On the Apps" Question (193)
#69 The Ex-Factor (194)
#70 Keeping on Your Best Behavior (195)
#71 Body Language, Eye Contact, and Those Active Listening Skills (197)
#72 Building Up Your Conversation Skills (198)
#73 Who Pays (202)
#74 How to End the Date Gracefully (203)
#75 Why You Might Not Want to Bother with Date 2 (205)
#76 Get Familiar with What Men Don't Want in Early Dating (207)
#77 Get Familiar with What Women Don't Want in Early Dating (209)
#78 Following Up Afterwards (211)
#79 Assessing the Connection (212)
#80 If You Had a Plain Weird First Date… Just Know You Aren't Alone (213)

chapter 7

FROM FIRST DATE TO SECOND... AND BEYOND

#81 Planning Date 2 (217)
#82 Mind Your Manners (218)
#83 Keep Multiple Dates in Rotation (219)
#84 The Block Hack (220)
#85 The 3-Date Barometer (220)
#86 Date 3 Complete? Red Flags to Be Aware of (221)
#87 How to Handle the First Month of Dating (225)
#88 Looking for This to Last Long-Term? More on What Not to Do (226)
#89 Keep the Momentum Alive (231)
#90 The Vacation Test: A Real-Life Reality Check (232)
#91 Signs It's All Moving Right (233)
#92 Signs It Is Time to Move On (236)
#93 Dodge the Dating Dilemmas (237)

chapter 8

GIFT GIVING 411

#94 Get to Know Your Dating Calendar (243)
#95 The Ins and Outs on Gift Giving (246)
#96 Thoughtfulness Speaks Volumes (247)
#97 The Big Gift-Giving Days… Valentine's (249)
#98 Don't Let Valentine's Day Derail You (250)
#99 Birthdays: A Day to Celebrate (253)
#100 Anniversaries: Keep It in Perspective (255)
#101 Just-Because Gifts (255)
#102 Rules of Thumb (256)
#103 Prepare Yourself for Summer Love (257)
#104 Unwrap the Holidays with Ease (260)
#105 Navigating the "New" in the Holiday Era (262)
#106 Launch into the New Year with a Dating Bang (264)
#107 Get Your New Year's Dating Mind Right (267)

chapter 9

DEALING WITH SETBACKS AND NEGATIVITY

#108 Handling Rejection and Moving Forward (271)
#109 Treasure Your Support System (272)
#110 Maintain an Upbeat Attitude (274)
#111 Phrases Confident Singles Use (275)
#112 How to Kick Your Dating Doubts to the Curb (278)
#113 How to Stay Positive When Dating
     Seems to Suck (280)
#114 Don't Slip Back into Divorce Regret (282)
#115 Responding to Criticism from Loved Ones (283)
#116 Reasons Why It May Not Be Working
     for You—Yet (284)

#117 Lessons Learned (285)
#118 Brutally Honest Reasons You're Still Single (287)
#119 A Roundup of Frequently Asked Questions (289)

chapter 10

ACHIEVING EXCLUSIVITY

#120 Having the "Exclusive" Conversation (293)
#121 To Bed and When to Bed (295)
#122 Take Care of the Buzz Kills (297)
#123 Not So Taboo Topics... Like STDs (299)
#124 Getting Down with the Sexy (300)
#125 Open to Experimentation (301)
#126 Scheduling Sex: To Plan or Not to Plan? (304)
#127 What Men Need to Make It Work (305)
#128 What Women Need to Make It Work (307)
#129 Looking at Labels (311)
#130 Tests, Quizzes, and Insights on Love Languages (314)
#131 Building Trust, Communication and a Shared Future (318)
#132 Clean Up the Camera Roll and Old Chats (320)
#133 Dealing with Social Media Use Dating and in a Relationship (323)
#134 Talk Money (327)
#135 More Tips for Lasting Relationships (337)

chapter 11

NAVIGATING FAMILY DYNAMICS

#136 Introducing a New Partner to Your Children (341)
#137 Balancing Dating and Family Responsibilities (343)
#138 Build a Supportive Family Environment (344)

chapter 12

SPECIAL CONSIDERATIONS WHEN DATING

#139 Dating as a Father or Mother to Children
    with Special Needs (347)
#140 Dating as a Widow or Widowers (349)
#141 Dealing with Past Divorces and
    Emotional Baggage (354)
#142 Finding Love After Major Life Changes (357)
#143 Adjusting to New Relationship Dynamics (360)

chapter 13

RECAP ON HOPE, LOVE, FUN— AND PREPARATION

#144 Make That Plan (363)
#145 Set Goals and Stay the Course (365)
#146 Constantly Innovate (368)
#147 Reminder: Get Out of Your Closed
    Mind Ways (369)

#148 Seek Out a Mentor (370)
#149 Pursue Professional Help When Needed (372)
#150 Hire a Dating Coach: A Strategic Investment (373)
#151 Celebrate Successes—Even the Small Ones (376)
#152 Continuously Improve You (377)
#153 Build High Self-Esteem (378)
#154 Prioritize Self-Care (379)
#155 Embrace Change (380)
#156 Fake It 'Til You Make It (381)
#157 People Aren't Always What They Seem (382)
#158 Great Writers Don't Always Write Great Messages (384)
#159 Maybe Your Kids Know More Than You About Dating? (385)
#160 Sometimes, Mom Knows Best (386)
#161 It Might Not Be a Rebound After All (387)
#162 Your Type Might Not Be Your Type (388)
#163 Bonus Tips from Golden Bachelor Contestant (389)
#164 Grit, Grit and More Grit (392)
#165 Embrace the Waves of the Marketplace (393)
#166 Remind Yourself: You've Got This (394)

ADDENDUM: WORKSHEETS #1-13 (395)
ACKNOWLEDGMENTS (411)

Disclaimer

The information provided in this book is for general informational and educational purposes only. While the author has made every effort to ensure the accuracy and reliability of the content, the book is not intended as a substitute for professional advice, therapy, or counseling. Readers are encouraged to seek the guidance of qualified professionals for any personal, medical, psychological, or financial concerns related to dating, relationships, or lifestyle choices.

The experiences and anecdotes shared are based on the author's personal and professional observations and may not apply universally to all readers. Dating and relationships are deeply personal, and individual experiences will vary. The author and publisher make no guarantees about the outcome of applying the ideas and strategies outlined in this book.

Readers should use their own judgment and discretion when implementing any advice provided. The author and publisher disclaim any liability for potential consequences resulting from the use or application of any information presented in this book.

33000 Dates Publishing

How to Use This Book

Welcome, Second Actor! I'm so glad you're here, taking the time to explore your path to new love and connection. As a "Second Actor," you're stepping into the dating world in your second half of life with intention, experience, and a refreshed vision of what you truly want and deserve. Whether you're single again or exploring love for the first time in a while, this second act is all about discovering what brings you joy, connection, and fulfillment. You've gained the wisdom of experience, and now, with a bit of guidance, it's time to apply that in exciting, purposeful ways.

There are two things you need to know in order to navigate *2nd Acts* successfully:

1. Each chapter is color-coded to represent a different phase of dating. These colors are part of the "rainbow ring" on the book cover designed to help you identify where you are in your journey, whether you're getting ready for dating, diving into digital matchmaking, or moving toward lasting connection.

Think of each section's color as a signpost guiding you through the phases of dating after 50. Each part provides the tools you'll need to navigate this new chapter, from taking care of yourself and understanding what you want to finding and building meaningful relationships.

2. Throughout this book, you'll find QR codes to be accessed by your smartphone, each code designed to bring an interactive element to your learning. Here's a quick guide to using them:

- **Turn on your camera.** Open the camera app—no need to take a picture! Just aim the camera at the QR code.

- **Frame the QR code.** Focus your camera on the QR code until a notification with a link appears on your screen.

- **Click the link.** It will direct you to the video. Watch the video and download the worksheet. Each worksheet is an essential step in your journey, designed to reinforce the principles and strategies in that chapter. Following the sequence and completing these worksheets in order will greatly enhance your experience, ensuring you're set up for success.

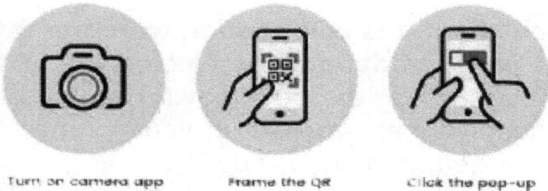

Turn on camera app   Frame the QR   Click the pop-up

ii

The QR Codes link to worksheets and videos that will dramatically help you on your way to dating. They are fun, interactive, and easily printable. You can also access them at the back of this book.

In this journey, take your time and immerse yourself in each chapter. These tools and insights are here to help you connect deeply and joyfully with yourself and others. My wish is that as you go through this book, you embrace your Second Act with a full heart and find love, companionship, and the fulfillment you deserve.

ANDREA MCGINTY | *2nd Acts,* Author

Click the QR code above for a message from Andrea McGinty to learn how to use this book!

chapter 1
How It All Began

(Hey, this is going to be quick, but stick with me as I want to show how it relates to you).

A Nostalgic Beginning: Family, Faith, and Aspiration in 1960s Cleveland

I was born in Cleveland, Ohio, in a 1960s world painted in pastel hues of tradition. My parents married in their early twenties and remained happily together until my mom, Maryann, passed away in 2002 at the tender age of 66. After her death, my dad Jack—also then in his sixties—ended up marrying his high school sweetheart. That's a whole story in itself and one I will dive into later in this book. (It's surprisingly common for people to rekindle old flames at high school reunions, just FYI.)

However, when we were a unit, we were that picturesque, nuclear model of familial love that sat around the dinner table every night. While Dad discussed serious issues like business and politics with Mom, my siblings and I goofed off, flicking our peas and pinching each other under the table. Yet I had big ears and loved to listen in, infatuated by their conversations on the retail business, business politics, and gossip about the Board of Directors.

We were also a Catholic family, devoted to the rituals of repentance and serving something higher than ourselves, and mass every week was a non-negotiable. But beyond the seriousness of our faith-fueled existence, I was the eldest of six kids, all born within a nine-year span.

With a massive extended family from both sides nearby, weekends and holidays were defined by dripping ice creams, endless shrieking through the suburban streets, and in my case, hitching up a frilly dress—always a baseball glove in hand or on the front-yard basketball court, always spattered with dirt, always reaching into the tentacles of my imagination, dreaming up all the places I would go and people I could be.

Nevertheless, our family's core values were clear: family, God, sports, and reading, led by the masculine archetype that was my father. Dad was a man of motion. Baseball and basketball were his playgrounds, but my earliest memories are of our backyard, a makeshift stadium where I was his eager fan and apprentice. I was his shadow from the tender age of four, learning to throw, swing, and volley. I also loved playing golf. Mom, surprisingly, was actually the golfing guru of our family—her gentle, feminine guidance shaping my swing. However, I embraced the notion of seasonal sports, following the rhythms inside the year: baseball in spring, basketball in winter, and volleyball in fall. This pattern forged a competitive spirit within me. Winning mattered; trophies were prized possessions, and I longed to fill the cabinets with gold-tinged figurines and my name emblazoned below each. That drive, born on the fields and courts where I first learned the thrill of victory, cemented itself into my brain and has never really let go.

My competitive drive wasn't just limited to sports. In everything I did, I wanted to—I had to—give my all. I was pretty type A, to say the least. Each year, I sold the most Girl Scout cookies of everyone in my class, by rushing off the school bus first and sprinting to the neighbors' homes before the other kids even had a chance to pull the change from their pockets.

Shaped by Strong Figures: A Father's Influence and a Mother's Example

I was especially close to my dad, who died in 2022. Jack was an amazing human being and a staunch advocate for women in the workplace. His influence shaped so much of who I am today, instilling in me the resolute belief that anything is possible. Dad grew up extremely poor yet emerged in life as the consummate self-made man. Starting as a stockboy at Higbee's, an upscale Ohio department store chain later acquired by Dillard's, Dad climbed the corporate ladder with unwavering dedication. He reached the position of President by the age of fifty. As one of the first three children, I experienced a middle-class upbringing. By the time the younger three arrived, Dad had established himself as a prominent figure in Cleveland's retail industry, ensuring they enjoyed a more financially secure childhood.

Meanwhile, my mom Maryann was the quintessential stay-at-home mom, managing everything on the home front. She had angel-soft hands and an ability to build beautiful meals from scratch, but I knew incredibly early on that such a domesticated, maternal route was not for me. I longed to be out in the wide world, working hard and making my own money.

Chasing Dreams and Testing Limits: Childhood and Adolescent Ambitions

Starting at the age of six, I jumped at the opportunity some weekends to accompany my dad to work at the department store, mesmerized by hundreds of flashing television screens flashing cartoons in the electronics department and the lingering scent of perfume sprayed by the sophisticated women sauntering through in their high-heels and elegant coats. Dad put me to work from 7 am until the shining twelve-story downtown store opened. My payment? A fancy lunch with him at the Silver Grille restaurant on the 11th Floor of Higbee's. I could not have been more thrilled.

Meanwhile, I was a super social child, to the point where a nun in third grade masking taped me to my desk so I wouldn't walk around and distract everyone with friendly conversation. Growing up, I was convinced I was destined for baseball stardom. The dream was so real that even my dad got caught up in the possibility. He took me to get my arm clocked—in other words, measured how fast I could throw.

Andrea McGinty

A good pitcher can consistently hit ninety miles per hour. I was a girl, so sixty-eight wasn't bad. Yet by the time I was fourteen, the harsh light of reality dawned on me. Major League Baseball, if we are going to be honest about it, wasn't in my future.

The Reality of Gender Roles: Growing up with Traditional Expectations

As I got closer to college age, my mother, who had studied nursing for two years but never finished, would remind me that college wasn't necessary for me the way it was for my brothers because it was their responsibility to raise and support a family. I suppose, in her mind, it would be a blessing to meet a good man who could take care of me. To her, I was the tall, skinny girl liked by the boys because of my athletic ability. That was the neat little path laid out before me: a path that did not feel like mine. I was not one of those whimsical teenagers fascinated with the fantasy of a big white wedding and Saturday afternoon strolls in the park with a toddler and a burgeoning belly. That whole spectacle of security and predictability felt like a nightmare. No, thank you. What I wanted more than anything was to live unencumbered, on the edge of everything, dancing until the early hours, meeting friends in stylish, dimly lit bars and building my life from the ground up.

But first, I needed to break hearts and sit with my own shattered heart a few times.

How It All Began

The Heartbreak and Lessons of First Loves

There was always something just a little wincing whenever I thought about boys—and I thought about boys a lot. The first thing I did when I turned sixteen was go on birth control. Of course, I could never tell my mother. This was the late 70s and early 80s, the fire and brimstone days of Catholicism. Our God wasn't this tender, forgiving, loving God you might have encountered at a non-denominational Church. Oh no. We went to mass on Sunday and then an extra day each week. Catholic guilt was heaped upon us at every turn, and we were warned of devastating consequences should we step out of line. I stepped out of line many times. However, that didn't mean I wasn't riddled with guilt when I did.

After high school, I attended a small Jesuit College named John Carroll University in University Heights, Ohio. The Jesuits are considered outliers and typically are not friends of the Pope. They do their own thing and have their own ideas. They believe that God can be found in every aspect of life, from nature to human relationships, are passionately committed to social justice and equality, and believe that education is a powerful tool for personal and societal growth. That's when I felt drawn back into faith and spirituality, relishing the opportunity to question, really question, life, love, and purpose.

Andrea McGinty

Throughout my first year, I dated Brett, who attended a different college not far away. He was Jewish, handsome, six foot two, and we met the summer between high school and college when he worked as a stock boy at Higbee's. Unfortunately, his family wanted him to marry a Jewish girl. After six months, the friction became too much, and we went our separate ways. Not long after, at age nineteen, I met who I thought then was the unabridged love of my life. Ace was in his sophomore year. He was a football player and avid athlete with enchanting brown eyes. He oozed charisma, lived life to the fullest and was exhilarating to be around.

For five years, we lived a romantic dream. By the time I graduated in 1984, our relationship was serious, but I was getting just as serious about my job search. The nation was recovering from the early 1980s recession caused by high inflation and interest rates, so the job market was especially tough, and I would toss and turn worrying about the next chapter. To the contrary, Ace shrugged his shoulders, undaunted by the struggles of the first world, and took off to ski on the slopes of Breckenridge, Colorado. I followed him for a short time, each day consisting of skiing and hanging out in the town, one day stretching into the next. I loved Ace, but I wasn't ready for marriage—for this to be all there was to my life. He wasn't ready either. It was time to find a job. A real job.

How It All Began

BIG DREAMS IN THE BIG CITY NEW YORK IN THE 1980S

It was 1985, and with my heart in my hand, I kissed my man goodbye and boarded a one-way flight for the Big Apple. Funnily enough, Ace—the free-spirited, ultra-cool skier—became a successful hedge fund manager.

Unlike Ace at this time, I had been in a hurry to figure it all out. Given my realization in high school that I would never be a baseball star, the next best thing when I entered college would be to aim for a lucrative career, taking Wall Street by storm. I was strong academically, although I did get easily bored and distracted—but I had taken accounting and finance classes in high school. Numbers came naturally. I reveled in the definitive nature of it: that there was a wrong and a right without the subjective interludes in between. I became a double major in accounting and finance. Mom begrudgingly agreed that this was the best route because "then you could do bookkeeping at home while you're pregnant" to help my husband out. I could only smile.

During college, I won an internship at Ernst and Young, one of the Big Four accounting firms. When I interviewed for a post-college position, the firm's chiefdoms had a different take.

The partner was gentle, yet his words cut deep.

Andrea McGinty

"You're smart," he conceded, "but this isn't for you."

They thought I was too bubbly, too brimming with energy for this kind of work, and feared I would quickly grow bored and quit. I was 22, and my world crashed down around me. At that moment, rejection felt like failure. Years later, I realized that the interviewer did me a favor. The corporate grind wasn't my destiny, and I sure as heck would have been bored out of my brain. My Wall Street dreams were officially over.

As a kid from Cleveland, the pulse of Manhattan in the mid-1980s was intoxicating, terrifying, incredible and empowering. By day, I followed in my father's footsteps and worked a retail job for 1928 Jewelry, which was—at the time—one of the top three most popular costume jewelry companies. I ran the accounts supplying department store behemoths Dayton's and Marshall Field's. By night, I waited tables at P.J. Clarke's, a famous American restaurant chain known for its classic comfort burgers and lively atmosphere, trying to afford the rent to my small apartment I shared with a bunch of other roommates on Central Park South. I danced and dated in the pockets of time in between, yet I couldn't keep up with the high-flying lifestyle of many of my peers who had voluptuous trust funds and inherited weekend homes in the Hamptons.

After about a year and a half of fun-fueled struggle, I decided time was up. The city's sheen had worn off, and I realized I needed a fresh start and a more affordable abode. In 1987, I stuffed my suitcase and headed to Chicago, where I already had a cadre of friends from my college days.

How It All Began

Redefining the Dream: Moving from New York to Chicago

The high-end neighborhoods of Lincoln Park and the Gold Coast became my new stomping grounds, and I continued my work with 1928 Jewelry. Then, I met *him,* the man I thought would be my forever. Mike was Black Irish, six-three, movie star good-looking and had made a name for himself in commercial real estate. Our eyes locked walking down the street, and from that moment onward, we shared three years of madness and magic. We became engaged, a milestone everyone in their mid-twenties was racing towards. I was caught up in the whirlwind, balancing love and dreams, and my Catholic roots that nagged at me to settle down and start a family.

Subsequently, I dipped my toes into the world of the woman I thought I would never be—the loser girlfriend, soon-to-be wife. I was motivated, but all my motivation was directed at Mike, trying to help him progress in his profession. I directed all my energy into his trajectory, offering suggestions and trying to boost his fragile ego. I also became the bride with glazed eyes who was fixated on ensuring I had the best set of China on the registry, planning for the perfect puffy gown, dreaming of the picket fence, and trying to decide on the number of children we would have and the square feet of our suburban home. I think, in retrospect, the social pressure of the time just got to me.

Andrea McGinty

Most of my college roommates were walking down the aisle, embarking on those grown-up married lives, and it felt like every other weekend I attended a wedding. At some point, I settled for this dream too, believing it was just the next step in life. I didn't know then what I know now: you can love people, you can understand people, but you can't change them.

Five weeks before the big day, Mike—out of the blue—said he had changed his mind. And that was that. I was shattered, the sort of fragmenting you think you can never pick yourself up and return from. But my devastation gradually winnowed as the months went by. Deep down, I knew it was never really going to work out. I wanted more for myself and wasn't ready to let that go in exchange for this tempered, conventional existence. There was something in me that wanted to set the globe on fire.

That break-up changed everything.

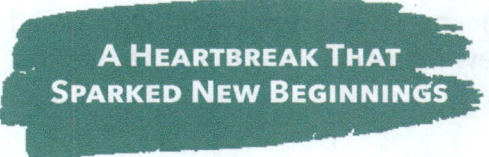

A Heartbreak That Sparked New Beginnings

My close girlfriends started to set me up. One had just graduated law school and was working in a large Chicago firm, teeming with eligible bachelors. They were dinner dates, which back then was the norm. Sometimes, that meant three or four elastic hours spent with someone you immediately knew just wasn't a fit.

How It All Began

I'm five foot nine, and more times than one, my blind date would be a guy who was maybe five, six or seven. Of course, there is absolutely nothing wrong with short men. However, it made me feel like this icky giant of a human being, and that wouldn't work.

After a little while, I concluded that my friends (bless their hearts) weren't particularly good at playing Cupid. I was exhausted, trying not to lose hope, but exhausted from the long, late and often awkward nights and the emotional toll the dating game took.

In the meantime, headhunters for the corporate arena were reaching out with opportunities, offering tempting positions in buying and other areas. But retail wasn't my calling, and the thought of returning to finance made me shudder. So, what was next? I needed a new career. And just as crucially, I needed some spark in my life away from work. I figured, *Why aren't there headhunters for people's personal lives?* I was 27 and would absolutely pay for someone to take time to fix me up with an individual who had similar interests or matched what I was ultimately looking for—and I knew I wasn't alone in those desires.

DATING CHALLENGES IN A PRE-DIGITAL ERA

An idea sparked: a personal life headhunter for people like me. Someone who could match people based on shared values, interests, and goals. I envisioned a cosmos where love was a science, not a gamble. That's when my next life chapter flew open—born from my own frustration with dating and the time devoted to what is often a losing cause. Never in a million years did I think I would ever be a professional matchmaker running a dating service. But actually, it wasn't all that far-fetched, and I wasn't a total rookie at this. After all, I fixed up one friend in high school who is still happily married and two friends from college. It was fun, unconventional, and a less traveled road that intrigued me.

Picture this: the dawn of the 1990s, pre-Google, pre-Amazon, pre-anyone being anything akin to computer savvy. Dating apps were a futuristic fantasy. So, there I was, open-eyed, armed with ambition and a yearning to change the game.

With zero business plan templates or online resources, I cobbled together a strategy in my mind. A friend of mine had just started the popular Italian restaurant concept Brio's and stressed to me that I needed a business plan and offered me his as a kind of template I could then develop into a structure. I came up with the company name "It's Just Lunch," abbreviated to IJL, but wanted to be sure I wasn't infringing on any existing trademarks. Unable to afford legal counsel, The Chicago Public Library became my war room, and the phone book my weapon as I prepped and plotted and scoured major cities to verify the name's availability. I then moved on to determine appropriate bars and restaurants that hosted "blind dates"—harmless, scheduled encounters over a quick drink where professionals could meet for an hour and decide if they wanted to go on a second date with that person. No more long and laborious dinners and time wasted trying to make conversation with someone that would go nowhere.

I showed my business plan to a few people, and the feedback was far from enthusiastic. My Irish twin brother Jim, who was just 11 months younger, married and working as a financial analyst, thought it was doomed to fail and said my numbers were too optimistic. He didn't believe there was a market for it. Another friend warned me about potential lawsuits, which I found confusing—what lawsuits? And yet another friend insisted that everything good had already been invented. I was frustrated by the constant negativity, so I decided to stop sharing my business plan. The lesson I learned was clear: if you strongly believe in something, go for it. Ignore the naysayers and the outside noise. I couldn't bear the thought of waking up at ninety, in a rocking chair, regretting that I never pursued the idea I had when I was in my twenties.

Only there was another glaring problem: no bank wanted to give me money. So, in 1991, I maxed out the $6000 limit on my credit card to get things up and running. I had to make it. There was no room for failure. There was no more money to spare. I worked seven days a week. And do you know what? I had a blast. Romantic relationships are the centerpiece of almost all our lives— the thing that takes up much of our thoughts and the thing that we want, perhaps more than anything else, to be successful, healthy and fulfilling. Playing such a pivotal role in people's lives felt incredibly rewarding.

My target: yuppies, the busy, urban professionals flooding Chicago's streets. They'd pay a fee to us pros running It's Just Lunch, and we'd handle everything from profiling to matching, and even restaurant reservations. The professionals on our roster would pay a set fee for a guaranteed number of setups that year.

First, they would come in for a one-hour interview, where I would get to know them and what they wanted, and from our internal pool, I could then start to schedule appropriate matches. I would only give each prospect a first name and a detailed description of their profession, back story, where they attended school, etc. But we would not show pictures nor disclose where they worked. Often, a little mystery is magic, and we didn't want people trying to track down their setup and develop an opinion about it before the meeting.

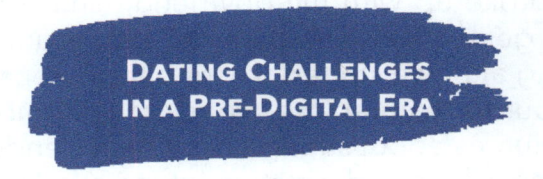

Dating Challenges in a Pre-Digital Era

After each scheduled date, we'd debrief with each prospect, gathering feedback about the other that would refine our matchmaking magic. Of course, the building blocks took time and It's Just Lunch started as a side hustle, and hustle it was. I spent weekends going door-to-door to clustered brownstone neighborhoods that house young, working professionals with my flyer in hand. I spotted a Chicago Tribune newspaper delivery guy doing his Sunday morning paper rounds in the exceedingly early hours of the morning and decided to tuck my flyers inside the paper. The paper boy couldn't care less what I was doing. It was a perfect advertising strategy, I told myself. The lesson here is to seize any opportunity, and it certainly was serendipity that I found him that night. Don't ask permission; ask forgiveness after the fact.

How It All Began

My flyers in the widely circulated Tribune gave people the impression It's Just Lunch had a lot of money, which meant credibility. I knew we would reach the perfect Sunday morning crowd—hungover and a little deflated at not having met anyone on their previous night's adventures. It didn't take long for the phone to ring. The voice on the other end was that of a young woman specializing in public relations. I had no idea what that was until Laura gave me the lowdown. This was 1990. We discussed marketing in college, but I had never heard of PR.

"I just broke up with my boyfriend," she explained. "So, you get me some dates, and I'll do your PR."

Not long after we started working together, the Wall Street Journal featured me in one of their quirky front-page columns about strange or offbeat trends. At the same time, a local radio station interviewed me about It's Just Lunch. The second my day job at 1928 Jewelry found out I was doing this on the side, they turned up their noses, and I was swiftly fired.

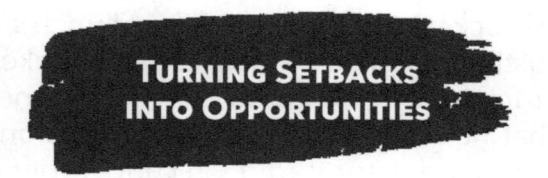

Turning Setbacks into Opportunities

At first, I was guttered. I distinctly remember standing in the grocery checkout line clutching my coupons, wondering if I were an idiot who would amount to nothing. I tried to wrap my head around how I would get the word out with no money for advertising and panicked about how I would make payroll. Trust me, there were so many times I teetered on the precipice of bankruptcy and almost lost it all.

Then, a woman tapped me on the back. Her name was Cheryl, and we had met the previous weekend. She asked me how the "dating thing" was going, and I put on my best and brightest smile and explained how one couple I had set up five or six months earlier had just gotten married. As it turned out, Cheryl was a producer at CNN and asked if she could do a segment, interviewing me and also following a couple out to lunch.

I knew that this was it, that I could not stray from the course when the going got tough. I had to give IJL my all. In addition to CNN, a few tiny articles led to prominent features, including Chicago Magazine and People Magazine. I had no money for advertising, but PR was a genius alternative.

About a year in, IJL took off like wildfire and I was able to hire a small team as devoted as I was to the cause. We meticulously researched cities, analyzing college education rates, income levels, and single demographics. Our target was clear: ambitious individuals seeking a more strategic approach to love. As our brochure boldly proclaimed, "It's time to take a professional look at your personal life." I moved us into a beautiful Chicago office space, but we could not limit ourselves to those walls, however gorgeous they were. It was time to expand; the most logical location was New York City.

Well, that was a freaking nightmare to get going. Nobody wanted to rent me office space, automatically assuming I was a madam like Heidi Fleiss. Even with the Wall Street Journal article in hand, the landlords dismissed me outright in that no-hold-barred New York City style.

How It All Began

Eventually, I found a spot on East 56th Street between 3rd and Lexington. The guy agreed to lease the space if I could pay the first year of rent upfront. Refusing to be deterred, I raced around acquiring loans from my dad and my grandma.

Then boom. The second location of It's Just Lunch was up and running. Soon, the knockoffs were up and running around the county, too. It was draining and stressful trying to distinguish myself from the potentially damaging "It's Only Lunch" or "What's Up For Lunch" businesses cropping up everywhere from Washington DC to Dallas, Texas, to Orange County, California. You can trademark a name, but you can't trademark an idea.

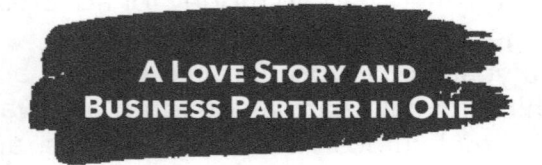

A Love Story and Business Partner in One

Nevertheless, It's Just Lunch was going from strength to strength as more couples found the loves of their lives. I was so busy I didn't expect love to fall into my own lap. I instituted a strict policy that employees were not allowed to date clients. That was an indispensable rule for the company's reputation and credibility. One afternoon in 1994, this dashing guy named Daniel walked into the Chicago office for an interview and promptly signed up for our services. He was a Harvard law graduate who specialized in Mergers and Acquisitions. I immediately thought of the incredible roster of women that would be perfect for him. However, Daniel called me immediately after.

"By the way," he said. "I came in just because I wanted to date you."

Naturally, I was flattered, yet politely explained that its policy is not to date with clients. Daniel wouldn't take no for an answer, emphasizing why we would make such a great match. Smiling graciously, I set Daniel up on his first date. The feedback I received from a talk show host, who said that the date was great, but he only talked about me. I shrugged it off and tried again. The next woman, Audrey, said the same thing. So, I called Daniel up to address it, reiterating that I wasn't on the market and that he needed to cut it out.

"Well, I want to go out with you," he persisted.

I reminded Daniel yet again that I do not date clients and do not overstep that boundary. A couple of hours later, he messengered over from his law firm a copy of the voided contract and a note explaining that he did not want a refund; he just wanted to take me out.

I sighed. One date, I figured. Well, we were married three months later, stayed married for 24 years, and had a daughter, Dagny, of our own. I suppose life happens when you don't always expect it. Yet in those initial months together, Daniel had just become a partner at his firm and was studying for his MBA. He offered to help me squash the growing cadre of knock-off companies.

"Why don't you just come work for me?" I suggested one day.

I believe the key to life is hiring smarter people than you. Daniel is an incredibly organized person, a trait that is not my forte. He understood money and how to talk to venture capitalists and private equity, and as CFO, he was immensely helpful in expanding It's Just Lunch across the country and the world.

The appeal of our model lay in its simplicity and efficiency, which was a breath of fresh air in the dating scene. At the time, there were no online dating options, and traditional matchmaking was almost non-existent outside of a few big cities like Los Angeles and New York. We offered a low-pressure, streamlined process where people could meet over lunch without the hassle of going to bars or relying on friends for introductions. Men appreciated not having to figure out how to meet women, and women liked not having to depend on their social circles or hope for organic encounters. The dating pool shrank as people reached their late twenties and thirties, making our straightforward approach even more attractive. Clients signed up for a year, and with each date, we got to know them better, refining our matchmaking process. Over a couple of years, we facilitated over 2000 marriages, proving the effectiveness of our method. Most dates were low-key lunches or after-work drinks, avoiding the pressure of lengthy dinner dates.

We needed capital to grow the company as we expanded into more markets. I approached eight different banks, and seven turned me down, but one banker saw the potential. He likened our model to the publishing industry and gave us a starter loan of a million dollars, which I paid back in a year. This initial success led to a larger loan of four to five million dollars, enabling us to roll out nationwide. With the new funds, we could afford advertising and PR efforts, becoming the largest advertiser in airline magazines. Our full-page ads in publications for airlines like Southwest, Delta, American, United, Singapore, and Emirates garnered national and international attention.

This visibility allowed us to expand into new markets like Singapore, Dublin, and beyond, solidifying our presence on a global scale.

The key lesson? Fake it until you make it.

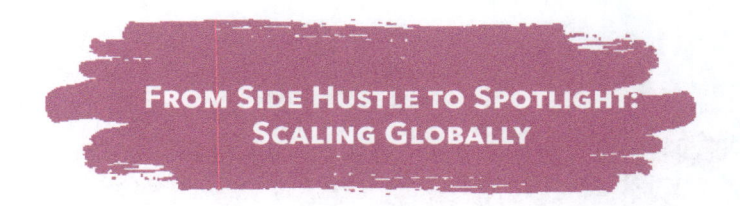

From Side Hustle to Spotlight: Scaling Globally

By 1997, our network spanned thirty U.S. cities from Minneapolis to Orlando, with our sights set on London, Paris, and Milan. Our projected earnings were a substantial $8-10 million, and we were catapulted into the spotlight when Oprah Winfrey invited me to share our unique story on her show. The media frenzy that ensued was overwhelming, and our Oprah appearance aired multiple times. It was a surreal journey from delivering brochures door-to-door to sharing our success on a global stage. Wow, we'd made it! Oprah. Who'd have thought a few years earlier I was putting brochures under people's doors?

Regarding the stigma of needing a matchmaker, I believe It's Just Lunch played a significant role in eradicating the negative perceptions around dating services. However, the real shocker was the tragedy of September 11. Although I rarely discuss this element, not wanting to seem opportunistic about such a catastrophic event, my business exploded in the aftermath. People shifted their focus from careers and money to loved ones and finding a partner, causing my business to more than double.

How It All Began

Before this, many mocked my company, dismissing it as a service for losers. I countered that it was actually for successful, busy people who worked hard on their careers and wanted guidance in their love lives. It's what smart people do—act.

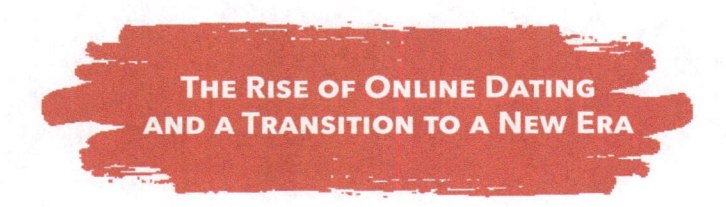

The Rise of Online Dating and a Transition to a New Era

Then, out of nowhere in 2009, the *Wall Street Journal* or an outlet of that caliber declared the dating space as hot for investors. Within a month, we had multiple calls from interested buyers. I hadn't seriously considered selling before, but with my daughter Dagny still young, the travel bug gnashed my brain. At this point, online dating was becoming more accepted, with about 1,400 sites out there. Some of them had really figured things out, offering a broader pool of people to meet than my model, which was based on physical locations like Chicago, each with around 1,000 members. Our very personalized model worked, but I could see the shift towards online platforms, with improved security and better user experiences. So, when offers started coming in (the executives from Match.com flew in on a private jet to chat, and private equity came knocking), I decided it was time. I was ready to sell and enjoy a more relaxed lifestyle. The decision to sell the company and transition to retirement was a reflective and contemplative one, marking the end of an era and the beginning of a new life phase.

Andrea McGinty

We had moved the headquarters to California by this point, splitting our time between Newport Beach and Palm Springs. Dagny was used to being on the move as we opened new markets, like spending a month in England to get a new location settled. It was fun and fulfilling, but I was ready for a change. The company had grown more corporate, with a board of directors and 700 employees. It wasn't like the early days of hustle and trying anything to make it work. It had to be formalized to succeed, however, that wasn't where my passion lay anymore. So, I accepted the deal from the private equity group and sold the company. With the sale, I was finally free to enjoy life, travel the earth, spend months in Morocco, Turkey, and China, and really do whatever I wanted.

Still, I knew deep down this wasn't my ultimate retirement plan.

Note to Reader

Of course, all client names, locations, and identifying details have been changed to protect privacy.

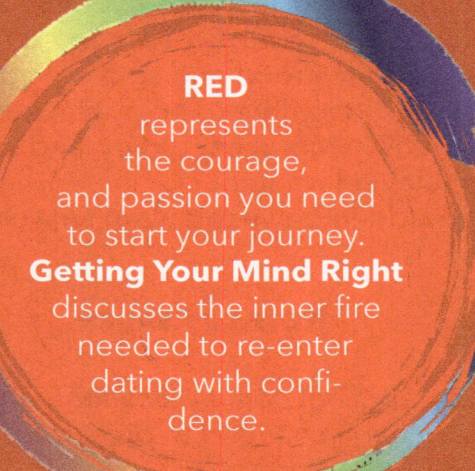

RED represents the courage, and passion you need to start your journey. **Getting Your Mind Right** discusses the inner fire needed to re-enter dating with confidence.

chapter 2
Getting Your Mind Right

*Red represents courage, passion, and
starting your 2nd-Act journey with confidence.*

#1 *Hire a Dating Expert*

The ah-ha moment for my next life chapter came in 2010 when I received a call from one of my best friends, Mark. Mark and his wife Sherry had amicably divorced two years before, which was wonderful for our friend group that we could stay friends with both of them.

**A FRIEND'S JOURNEY AND
AN EYE-OPENING REVELATION**

So, when Mark hit his late forties, newly divorced in Southern California, I was his go-to confidante. His tales of online dating woes were endless—from women who looked nothing like their pictures to supposed high-profile careerists who were, in fact, unemployed.

With a growing despair, Mark was convinced the early digital dating scene was a wasteland, yet seemed to have no idea how to introduce himself online, where to go, or how to present himself on a first or second date.

Mark is an intelligent guy (a CFO for a well-known company) and if he was clueless about this, then it was a good bet there were *many* more smart folks out there just as overwhelmed and confused. I listened diligently, but my playing passive wasn't serving him.

One afternoon, exasperated with Mark's latest dating disaster, I blurted out, "Give me your login. I'll take a look." Hesitantly, he handed over his credentials. What followed was a cringe-inducing quest through a digital profile that screamed "desperate and green." Think shirtless selfies, generic platitudes, and a complete lack of personality were a recipe for online dating disaster.

I went to work, deleting cringe-worthy photos, crafting a compelling bio, and selecting images that showcased Mark's personality and success. A few weeks later, Mark called, his voice filled with excitement and disbelief.

"I've been on the best dates ever! These women are amazing," he enthused.

It didn't take Mark long to find his first post-divorce love, and he shared with friends how much my guidance helped. Those friends subsequently reached out for some help, and then, the next thing you know, friends of friends were trying to get in touch. All of a sudden, I was the default personalized dating consultant for online dating.

A light bulb went off.

From Casual Support to a Professional Business

What started as a favor for Mark quickly turned into a full-blown business, primarily from word of mouth, that I enjoyed and, if I say so myself, was rather good at. I named my next venture "33,000 Dates," a nod to the number of dates I had set up during my time running It's Just Lunch. Soon, some of the clients I had worked with in my former business were also seeking services, but now they were older, coming out of marriages and long-term relationships, their kids were well past the diaper days, and they were ready for the next epoch of their personal lives.

I, too, was in the twilight of my late forties and could relate to just how intense digital dating could be to someone used to meeting the person of their dreams "out in the wild." But the world had dramatically changed for these once powerhouse twenty or thirty-somethings on the ITJ Rolodex, and they weren't quite sure where to begin. The upside is that by hiring an expert, they didn't have to start from scratch. The key is having someone by your side, an advocate, who can put you on the highway to success from the get-go.

Turning Life Experience into Expertise

Your career trajectory was not simply fate: you had a plan. Why not opt for a similar strategy regarding your personal life, too?

And just like you hire a mechanic to fix your broken-down vehicle, a hairdresser to cut your hair, or a coach to teach you a golf swing for the first time, dating deserves some expert elevation. Doing everything yourself isn't wise. Enlisting a pro in your court will save you time, money, energy and heartache in the long run. There are thousands of dating sites and apps and many thousand more opinions on what works and what does not. Let someone who knows their stuff take the guesswork out of this.

"Online dating is like going into an unknown jungle with all kinds of wild animals, dangerous plants, and traps… but also gorgeous flowers, sweet animals and revitalizing pools. Andrea is the no-nonsense safety guide who does the briefing BEFORE you go in and then is also the guide who points out things along the way," one of my client's wrote. *"Sometimes, she has to pick you up after a bad fall and dust you off. Now, imagine going into the jungle with NO guide or briefing…. no wonder people have horrible experiences!"* Quote from Chrissy, 52, a client in NYC.

But how do you find the right dating expert, and what should you expect? Here's a breakdown of the critical things to consider before hiring:

9 Key Moves to Make Before You Hire a Dating Coach

1. Experience is Everything. Look for a coach with a proven record. They shouldn't just have met their spouse online; they should have helped **thousands** of clients find love. Ten to fifteen years of experience is a good benchmark. This ensures they've seen the evolution of online dating platforms and can adapt to the latest trends.

2. Know Your Niche. Choose a coach who understands and caters to your age group or demographic. Ideal suitors for a 55-year-old man are unlikely to be the same as those for a 20-something.

3. Clear Communication is Key. Beware of coaches without a phone number. This could be a red flag for a ghostwriter or someone unreliable. Consistent communication is crucial for a successful coaching experience.

4. Transparency Builds Trust. Pricing should be clearly outlined on the coach's website. Avoid situations where pricing feels undefined or negotiable.

5. Profile Powerhouse. Look for a coach who will rewrite your profile from scratch. Being objective about yourself is hard, but a pro can concoct a compelling bio that attracts the right matches. Revisions after the initial draft are paramount. Aim for a turnaround time of 48-72 hours.

6. Picture Perfect. The right photos are critical. Your coach should be skilled at choosing and optimizing images that showcase your personality and best qualities.

7. Strategic Selection, Not Blind Casting. Avoid coaches who recommend trying every dating app or platform. This scattershot approach is ineffective. Look for someone who can research your demographics and geographical area to recommend the most suitable sites.

Getting Your Mind Right

8. Success is a Journey. Understand that no coach can guarantee a happily ever after. However, their guidance can significantly increase your chances.. Aim for a coach with a success rate of around 50% (dating someone they genuinely like).

9. Dating Should Be Fun! Choose a coach who makes dating an adventure, not a chore. They should be encouraging and supportive and help you refine your approach along the way.

WORKSHEET #1—
How to Rate a Dating Coach

ALERT! The QR code above will take you to a short video from Andrea with more on this topic plus a downloadable worksheet.

#2 Be Sure You Are Ready... to Go All in

Before you invest in a professional or use this book as your expert guide to plunge back into the game, you want to be sure you're ready—really ready. This isn't an endeavor for the half-hearted. For this to work, you must be willing to put in the hard yards, get comfortable with being uncomfortable, and not run if the going gets tough.

Andrea McGinty

Ready to Date? A Real Decision

Re-entering the dating pool is a decision. But it is critical to ask yourself some questions first, which will determine your level of success.

I'll give a personal example. I was divorced in 2018 after a 24-year marriage. Was I ready to date?

Heck, NO! And that is despite the decades spent matchmaking and bolstering others in the love and confidence arena.

My life was in transition: moving from the big house to a new condo, my daughter in her early teens, and I couldn't fathom adding dating to this confused tableau. My daughter was the priority and was in very formative years. Imagine throwing in a mom dating a slew of men to the picture. It just felt, well, not right. Stability was my goal, and I learned who I was alone. Plus, I knew that my time on the West Coast was numbered, with my daughter growing up and planning to venture to the East Coast for college.

Fast forward five years. My youngest was now a senior in high school and busy with her life. And just like that, I woke up one morning and declared to myself, "It's time; I'm ready to date." For those of you with whom I am fortunate to work, you know me, and I jump enthusiastically into things. That day, I wrote my profile (no, I still don't recommend you all writing your own!), went with the first draft (for you all, I am a bit nuts and revise four times minimum before sharing with you), looked through my photos, called my best friend's husband (a professional photographer), and asked him for an hour to shoot a few new photos to mix with my iPhone and Instagram photos. Yes, I was off to the races in less than a week.

DIVING IN: THE 5-DATE WEEK

As someone allergic to procrastination with no patience to mess around, I identified the two sites I wanted to begin with, and *boom*— I'm on. The following week, *ta-da,* I have 5 dates. Yes, 5. My stomach churns just thinking about this again. I reached out to 5 different men and limited our conversation to just a couple of messages before I suggested meeting up for lunch. (Yes, of course, I'm not a dating site magician. I wrote to 25 men, and only 5 got back to me—so pretty standard odds). Still, I went through all the pangs everyone in the dating game endures in their minds. A couple of extremely cute, accomplished men never responded, and I wondered why.

Nevertheless, I quickly shut down those thoughts (who the heck knows why they didn't get back to me?) and moved on positively to those who did. There is no time to dwell in digital dating. Focus on the upside.

5 Dates. 7 Days. I drew a deep breath. With all I know now, I don't recommend this, but my enthusiasm and go-go attitude got me in this pickle. Admittedly, the dates were lovely even if they didn't entail Mister Forever. I was offered a window into the lives of some remarkably interesting men, and was reminded that I could still have conversations and be somewhat charming even after all those years away from singledom. My dating skills were still there, just a bit rusty.

1. Date 1: A hedge fund guy. It was totally polite, though we both knew no chemistry. The outcome? He invited me several weeks later to this dinner affiliated with *Shark Tank* producers, and I met some interesting people and contacts for later business endeavors.

2. Date 2: Drummer in a rock and roll band. OMG. This guy was gorgeous, so out of my wheelhouse of what I wanted at the time, but so much fun with such an uplifting vibe.

3. Date 3: A Podcaster. The conversation totally rocked. However, the chemistry was nowhere to be found. Still, the guy has a full studio and invited me to use it anytime it was free. Such a nice human!

4. Date 4: Entrepreneur type. We bonded over both having lived in Chicago, and we went on three dates before it fizzled. (Wow, I can still get a second and third date—yay, me!) My confidence bloomed, and sometimes, that's the biggest coup when returning to the pool.

5. Date 5: A doctor. We had nothing in common, so I sat quietly and listened to him discuss the latest skincare and vitamin therapy advances. I learned quite a bit from him; it was like a free consultation and time well spent!

Despite the positive experiences, I was exhausted after that week, plus I couldn't remember what I talked about with each person. You don't want to look flaky on a second date repeating a story over again, right? So do as I say, not as I do. Pace matters.

I took a break. That meant two weeks to see how a few second dates would go.

Yet there was still this one mystery man I hadn't met. Jeff lived near me in South Florida but messaged me he was up at the Cape for a few weeks. I was drawn to him because his message read, "You know what impressed me most about you? That you host Thanksgiving yearly for family and friends and do all the cooking yourself for 40 people. Wow!" That compliment melted my heart. Jeff wasn't impressed by anything I'd done business-wise. Instead, he got to the heart of something I care tremendously about: family and friends. It felt like one of those rare incidences where somebody doesn't just look at you, but they see you.

Jeff and I never talked on the phone. We just met for lunch and *boom*—I really liked him. When I initially met him, I stuck out my hand to shake his. We laughed and chatted. Then, when the date ended, he shook my hand. I thought, *Oh, no, he doesn't like me.* (All the other dates had hugged me). But the rest was history, and a year later, here we sit, a solid couple, chemistry, love, and best friend with whom I have a blast! And it turns out our first date was on his birthday. So on July 21, we celebrated two milestones—him and us. By the way, we're married now.

TOP TEN QUESTIONS BEFORE YOU BEGIN DATING AGAIN

So here are the TOP TEN questions you should ask yourself before jumping into dating—whether online dating, matchmaking, speed dating, or hiring an expensive one-on-one matchmaker. I would encourage you to use the worksheets in this book especially dedicated to your personal expedition and dating adventures. I love handwriting because it forces us to connect with ourselves in a very primal way, without the technological disconnect.

While I am passionate about helping singles of all types and stripes find love, and my expertise spans all age groups, this book focuses on the 2nd Acts crowd, primarily those aged 40s to 60s. The anecdotes, advice and lessons apply to all relationships, including heterosexual, homosexual, bisexual, transgender, and lesbian. We all seek love or companionship, and while my coaching has primarily centered on heterosexual relationships, I'm grateful for the internet's ability to connect people of all orientations.

WORKSHEET #2— AM I READY TO START DATING AGAIN?

(I offer free 15-minute consultations to assess your readiness. I'm honest about whether I can help you and why if not. If you're seeking love or simply want to date again, let's chat. But in the interim, let me guide you through this book and propel you into the best shape possible for this wonderful new era of your life. I promise you, if you can stick it out and give it everything you have to give, it will work out.)

#3 Attitude Is Everything

BREAKING THE MYTH: "ALL THE GOOD ONES ARE TAKEN"

One of the biggest hurdles people face when re-entering the dating world is the pervasive belief that "all the good ones are taken." Men often say, "All the great women are already in relationships." While women say, "All the amazing men are already married." This is a limiting mindset that can stifle enthusiasm and hinder progress. It's also false. The truth is that there are countless amazing people out there looking for meaningful connections, and dating after 45 can be an incredibly liberating experience, ushering you into a whole new lease on life.

Let's look at the facts. According to the Pew Research Center, more than 28% of the U.S. population between 45 and 65 are single. An even more sizable portion of those individuals—more than 30%—actively use dating platforms. That's a heck of a lot of people. The numbers don't lie. A vibrant and active dating community exists, and there are many special souls waiting to be found.

Shifting to an Abundance Mindset

I can't help but laugh and reflect on the frequent calls I receive from my clients who have found their someone after sifting through the initial self-doubt and worry that there were no "good" ones left. I think I have the most incredible job in existence, but you have to believe that love again is possible and be ready to recognize Mr. or Mrs. Right when they arrive.
Instead of fixating on scarcity, shift your focus to abundance—approach dating with a strategic mindset. Just like any successful endeavor, dating requires a plan. It's not about aimlessly browsing through profiles but identifying compatible partners and engaging in meaningful interactions. You're not searching for a needle in a haystack; you're looking for a specific type of person who aligns with your values and goals.
Throughout this journey, maintaining a positive attitude is key. First up, surround yourself with supportive friends. Like a workout buddy, having someone to share your experiences can boost your motivation and help you stay focused. A positive mindset can make a significant difference in your dating experience.

Staying Positive and Persistent

Be patient and persistent. Not every date will be a perfect match, but each interaction is an opportunity to learn and grow. Celebrate small victories, no matter how insignificant they may seem. Finding love is a marathon, not a sprint.

Adopting a positive, initiative-taking approach will increase your chances of finding a fulfilling relationship. Trust in the process, believe in yourself, and enjoy the trek—you never know where you will end up. Consider this: you don't have to rely on bars to meet people. You can effectively use dating platforms with the right strategy and a targeted approach. It's not about aimlessly scrolling; it's about having a plan for each interaction.

Your attitude is everything and it will make or break you in the dating world.

#4 Embrace the Unique Challenges of Dating after 50

There's a common misconception that dating after 50 is awkward, embarrassing, or a sign of failure. This couldn't be further from the truth. Your 50s are an exciting time to embark on a new epoch of your love life. Sure, it is natural for humans to feel apprehensive about trying new things. Consider the first time you stepped onto a pickleball court, thinking, "This is so popular. What if I'm terrible at it?" However, chances are you didn't let that stop you. You probably attended a clinic, learned the rules, had some fun, met new people, and realized that pickleball combines ping pong and tennis, and yes, it was enjoyable! Your anxiety disappeared, and a new passion was born.

Breaking the Myth of Scarcity: Amazing Matches Do Exist

Long gone are the days when online dating was considered taboo. Today, it's a mainstream way for people of all ages and walks of life to connect. That silly stigma of "it must be for people who can't score in the real world" is rapidly fading. It's rare to meet the next love of your life in the wild and if you are still clinging to that storied fable, it is time to let it go. Digital dating allows you to cut out the BS and a lot of what you don't want before you spend precious time and provides you with a smorgasbord of hope and possibility from the comfort of your couch.

Look at digital dating as a way to leverage technology and expand your social circle, meeting people who share your interests. For instance, online dating can introduce you to a wider range of potential partners than you might meet in your daily life and provide a platform for meaningful conversations and connections.

By your 40s and 50s, you've experienced much of life. You know who you are, what you value, and what you want in a partner. This clarity lets you be more selective and intentional in your dating pursuits. We understand that life throws unexpected curveballs. Maybe you're divorced, widowed, or simply ready for a fresh start. Dating after 50 is about embracing the opportunity to find love and companionship on your own terms.

I have helped set up over 33,000 dates, and along the way, I have heard countless stories, excuses, fears, and frustrations. My experience has given me unique insights into the domain of dating, and I'm here to share that knowledge with you.

Here's what I frequently hear from frightened or misinformed daters—and why, in general, they are wrong. (And they find this out fairly quickly!)

8 Common (but Misinformed) Objections to Online Dating

1. There is a stigma associated with online dating. The self-talk goes something like this: "I must be desperate. How could my love life have come to this? The internet is full of scary men/women whose intentions are dishonest." Truth: With the advent of online dating in the 90s came utter chaos: the internet, Google, and dating sites were in their infancy. While it took about 20 years, many online sites and apps have done an excellent job setting up fail-safe procedures and verifications. Where did this get us? To a widely accepted method of dating.

2. You were married in your 20s or 30s before online dating became prevalent. You may reminisce about the ease and naturalness of dating in your 20s or 30s before online dating became prevalent. You recall many potential partners you encountered through college, grad school, and the workplace, where face-to-face interactions were a daily occurrence. Organic, right? Let's not forget it wasn't exactly easy then, either.

You had to schlep to bar after bar or from one blind date to another. It was kind of like childbirth—hurts like hell, but a week later you forget the pain. Well, things have changed. Online dating is not necessarily easier or harder; it's just different. But new is daunting, I get it. At 55 or 60, divorced, and with no prior experience in online dating, it is only natural to feel nervous about trying an innovative approach. You aren't alone, my friend.

3. Everyone brings baggage to the relationship. I don't think of it this way. Everyone brings their own life experiences to the table. It's all about perspective—these experiences shape who you are today. Dating after 50 may come with its own set of challenges, like dealing with children and ex-spouses, but it's also an opportunity to enrich your life with new experiences and new people to love; sometimes more than one! In meeting my second husband, I also became a stepmom to more children who I just adore and now I cannot imagine my life without them. You never know what excitement is around the corner.

4. You are afraid of what people will think. You are frightened by the idea that friends or family (or even your kids) may see you online. That was a fear I saw among clients in the early 2000s, but now it has become a widely accepted dating method. (And chances are that those critics are probably—secretly—online, too!)

5. You have read many horror stories in the media about online dating. You may fear stalkers and gold diggers or being taken advantage of. Of course, with hundreds of thousands of people online and over 1400 dating sites and apps out in cyberspace, there will be some. Fortunately, it's 2025, and while they have not been completely eradicated, they are rarer. Who can forget the Nigerian prince asking for money (a big scam in its day)? Or a posing prospective love interest asking for money for a plane ticket to visit you? The media has done a decent job educating us on the pitfalls of online dating, but bear in mind the press is also looking for sensationalist and unique stories: *exceptions*. We are too well-educated about online dating now to fall for these types of scams, and online sites/apps have features to identify and remove these issues. (See tips on how to avoid scams in Chapter 4).

6. Online dating is visual. Yes, this makes the average person nervous. The fear of rejection based on looks alone is typical. However, with the forthcoming tips in this book, we will make sure your photos illuminate the best of you—in and out.

7. Most of your friends are married but don't understand your situation. How often have you heard them say, "I know this amazing guy who would be perfect for you! You don't need to resort to online dating." And how often does that setup actually happen? The reality is, when it comes to dating, your married friends are not the best advisors. (Even your single friends can be unhelpful if they have a negative mindset). If this is the case, keeping your online endeavors close to the chest until you're ready to surprise your friends by bringing your new "friend" to a dinner party is best.

8. There is a common perception that online dating is only for the younger crowd. This is no longer the case. While the 20s and 30s may be using Tinder, that doesn't mean you have to. Numerous dating sites are specifically designed for the 50+ age group, and choosing the right one is important for success. You want to be on a platform that caters to your demographic, has a strong presence in your geographical area, and offers a higher percentage of potential matches of a different sex. For example, I have a 56-year-old client, Reese, an executive at Google in California, who was unhappy with online dating when he came to me. A friend in New York City had recommended Coffee Meets Bagel. While this may be a strong choice for the East Coast, its membership is minimal out West. Once on the right site, Reese began meeting quality women. (More on that coming right up!)

#5 Remind Yourself That There Are 3 Ways to Approach Dating

1. The Adventure Approach. This is the optimal approach, whether or not you're new to online dating. Adventure brings excitement, but it can also stir up a bit of nervousness, which is completely normal when trying something new or even scary! Here's what one client said about online dating with a dating coach: "Working with Andrea was a fantastic experience. Her extensive knowledge and experience made her an invaluable asset. She was like a canary in a coal mine, always able to anticipate potential issues and save me time and effort!"

2. Whiner Approach. Uh-oh, the title gives away how this approach usually ends. Not well, right? Unfortunately, I see this attitude from time to time. Where does it come from? Let's list some possibilities and see if any of these sound familiar:

- You tried online dating once (half-heartedly) and got no responses,

- You sent a few hearts or likes but didn't follow up with a message, leaving men frustrated (this is their number one complaint),

- You wonder why an accomplished, good-looking person would even need online dating,

- You've heard horror stories about dating sites or apps from single friends,

- You call me with preconceived notions that there are no good men left, or

- You believe all the good ones are married.

 It's time to adjust your mindset. These might have been valid concerns in the 90s and early 2000s, but online dating has changed dramatically. Your attitude needs to shift to at least a neutral—if not positive—outlook. Consider the following:

- 48% of Americans are single, according to the US Census Bureau,

- There are over 1,400 dating sites/apps in the US, and

- The number one way people in their 50s-70s find relationships is through online dating.

To be blunt, if you were divorced, widowed, or single in the 1990s, meeting the right people at our age would have been tough—not anymore. We are so fortunate!

So, how do I handle a whiner client? Take Laura, 62. I immediately advised her to stop talking to her negative, single friends about dating. Instead, she started consulting an impartial third party, a good dating coach, to help keep her spirits up and maintain perspective.

The Challenge Approach

I really like this one! My female clients often decide to open their hearts and minds for a three-month period and give online dating their all. Why does this work?

- It's for a short, manageable period.

- They commit fully.

- They invest in professional photos (and no, these don't have to be expensive—I work with resources that charge $200-$250, and it's a worthwhile investment).

- Like taking up yoga, golf or pickleball, they seek expert help to navigate the process.

- They trim down their list of must-haves to 2-3 essentials (such as religion, geography, education level, etc.).

- When they find an interesting man online, they don't wait for him to make the first move—they send a fun, informative message expressing interest.

- During the first two weeks, they go on 4-5 first dates. Yes, really! It's like going to the gym—by date five, you'll be more practiced and comfortable.

Tara, 58, was initially uncomfortable sending messages. Back in November, her typical message was just a heart with "Hi, how are you?" Unsurprisingly, this generic approach got zero responses because it came across as uninterested and lazy. Since then, Tara has graduated to sending 2-3 sentence messages that show she read the dating profile and has genuine interest. By February, she went on six dates, and my fingers are crossed for Tara!

Attitude is everything, and yes, I see people fall in love every month—sometimes every week. That's why I do what I do!

A mix of red's intensity and orange's warmth, **VERMILLION** symbolizes self-expression and uniqueness which are critical for **Building Your Brand.**

chapter 3
Building Your Brand

#6 Take a Business-Minded Approach

THE BUILDING BLOCKS: PLANNING, RESILIENCE, AND SELF-AWARENESS

Starting a business and building a relationship share striking similarities. Both ventures require a leap of faith, strategic planning, and resilience. Just as a startup seeks that idea-saving investment, a relationship often hinges on finding the right partner. Like navigating a business, couples must make joint decisions, manage shared resources, and maintain open communication. Both journeys are filled with trial and error, and the importance of self-awareness cannot be overstated. While external advice is abundant success lies in understanding one's strengths and weaknesses, and persistently pursuing long-term goals.

OVERCOMING COMMON PITFALLS: COMMITMENT AND CONSISTENCY

In both business and relationships, common pitfalls can hinder progress. Inadequate planning, a lack of understanding about the market or partner, and a reluctance to seek assistance are frequent obstacles. By prioritizing organization, curiosity, and unwavering commitment, we can overcome these challenges. Recognizing the parallels between these two endeavors offers valuable insights into fostering success in both personal and professional life.

In an Andrea-esque nutshell? Have a plan. Do the legwork. Put yourself out there. Reap the rewards, with the expectation that returns are not necessarily a linear progression or happen from the get-go. Some startups can get lucky, but most require a good amount of blood, sweat and tears.

#7 Put Work into Personal Branding

Clever personal branding is the secret sauce to stand out in the crowded online dating world. Most profiles blend together, offering generic lists of interests and preferences. That's boring and isn't going to grab anyone's attention. Instead, think of your profile as an artfully constructed brand identity. You want to be unforgettable for all the right reasons.

By displaying your unique qualities and values, you create a compelling narrative that resonates with potential matches. Just like a successful business, your personal brand should be memorable, consistent, and authentic. A personal brand is your story and how you present yourself. It demonstrates your unique qualities and skills. You need to stand out in the dating macrocosm—and your brand will lead the way.

Avoid the Vanilla Profile Trap

The problem? Most online daters fall into the trap of generic profiles. They list places they've traveled, hobbies they enjoy, or the must-have qualities in a partner. This bland approach is, quite frankly, a snooze fest.

WORKSHEET #3—
Craft Your Narrative with Personal Branding Brainstorm

Imagine your profile as a story about you! Use strong visuals and spellbinding text to highlight your personality, interests, and values. What makes you tick? What are you enthusiastic about? This personal branding strategy will help you connect with potential matches who share your interests and outlook on life. Give us some swagger, some edge, something that makes you the most intriguing person in the room.

BORROW FROM BUSINESS BRANDING

Think of the successful brands you know. What makes them memorable? They have a clear, consistent message. Apply this concept to your profile. Develop a short, impactful tagline that summarizes your unique essence. Keep it brief, like the slogans of major companies. This tagline will be your personal branding statement in the dating world.

One client, a 42-year-old writer and global traveler living in New York City used the catchy "Flower Child with a Rock n' Roll Soul," which—without having to say more—conveyed her essence as a calm, crunchy mama with a perchance for a fun time. So, get your creative cap on.

#8 Take Time Out to Develop Your Story

Defining Your Unique Brand: The Key to Online Dating Success

Developing a strong personal brand is the fundamental building block for navigating the competitive world of online dating before you begin the process. By clearly defining your values, skills, and unique qualities, you'll attract like-minded individuals and boost your confidence. A well-conceived personal brand sets you apart from the crowd, allowing your authentic self to shine through. Whether you're a science enthusiast or a fashion-forward individual, embracing your unique personality is key to creating a compelling online presence.

Stand Out and Shine: Creating a Compelling Online Presence

What makes you stand out? What are you passionate about? Clearly defining your brand will help you create a profile that resonates with potential matches. Just like a well-designed magazine, keep your online profile concise and impactful. For one, I had one client who was 53 and really into Formula One. Not only was she an avid spectator, but she knew how to race and pull the car apart and put it back together with greasy hands. What guy wouldn't want to take a look at this pretty stand-out woman?

Building Your Brand

WORKSHEET #4—
PLOTTING YOUR SELF-REINVENTION

When entering the Second Act world of dating, you must do a "rebranding" from what you've been for the past 20 or 30 years. Maybe you were a stay-at-home Mom, a singleton with tunnel vision on your career, or a man recently widowed after a treasured 30-year marriage.

Time to reinvent yourself without sacrificing your authenticity? Yes! I highly encourage this! Questions to ask yourself, and you can write the answers below.

#9 Turning to Your Friends

To define our skills, value and hot selling points clearly, I strongly suggest enlisting the help of those who know us best to get it right. We can overlook things or forget how the external world sometimes sees us. Bringing to life a compelling personal brand requires a fresh perspective. So, call on your closest friends and family to help you define your unique selling points. This outside perspective can uncover hidden strengths and create a captivating narrative.

Getting Perspective from Family and Friends

I have my clients text—do not call—asking five close friends or family members to describe you in five words and share anecdotes that highlight your personality. Give those chosen few the chance to think about it. I don't want these to be generic descriptions like fun, good sense of humor or kind. These don't really tell us about you. Urge them to go deeper and tell us why they use these descriptors.

And just to reiterate why this is so important, I once had a client who was a multiple times New York Times bestselling author, one of the most esteemed writers on the planet. Yet, he could not write a dating profile or create an interesting elevator if his life depended on it. You would have thought the man was a glorified plumber if you read what he put together. While there is certainly nothing wrong with plumbers, his profile failed to capture who he was and what he had to offer.

Bottom line: we need outside counsel to get this right.

Choosing the Right Words

In the world of online dating, your profile is your first impression, and the words you choose can make all the difference. That's why I have created a guide to help you elevate your language from BORING to GOOD, and ultimately to GREAT.

- BORING words often fall flat, failing to capture your unique personality.

- GOOD words get closer—they may hint at who you are but lack the flair to make you memorable.

- GREAT words, however, bring your profile to life. They resonate with authenticity, spark curiosity, and make potential matches pause and want to learn more.

  By aiming for GREAT, you're not only showing your best self but also setting the stage for meaningful, lasting connections. In online dating, great words are more than just vocabulary—they're your personal brand. On the next page, I have listed some suggestions

Boring, Good, OR Great?

BORING

kind-sense of humor-happy-positive-romantic-active-loving-intelligent-curious-passionate (so overused)-soulmate-authentic-generous-mindful-crazy-blunt-polite-interesting-warm-tough-timid-cultured-honest-caring-spontaneous-happy

GOOD

athletic-nurturing-playful-thoughtful-pragmatic-appreciative-engaged and plugged in-wise-frugal-**self-sufficient**-financially stable-compassionate-humble-**easy going**-accomplished-ambitious-creative-**kindhearted**-empathetic-calm-diplomatic-conservative-liberal-**warm-hearted**-savvy

GREAT

quirky (but describe how)-nerdy-bookish-chill-exuberant-explorer-**big-hearted**-witty-**self-deprecating**-analytical-artistic-introverted-extroverted-eccentric-dynamic-affectionate-**down-to-earth**-tech savvy-**soft-spoken**-imaginative-**community-minded**-inventive-independent-physically fit-perceptive-sweet

33000Dates.com

#10 Crafting the Dating Elevator Pitch

Every remarkable story starts with an engaging opening. Your online dating profile is no different. A strong headline, often called an "elevator pitch" in the business world, is essential for grabbing attention. It should be concise, engaging, and reflective of your personality. Many people shy away from writing headlines, fearing they might sound boastful. Don't let this deter you! Remember the business plan. Businesses do not succeed in playing shy or downplaying what they have to offer. With a bit of creativity, you can bring to life a headline that perfectly sets the stage for the rest of your profile.

Your Elevator Pitch

Once you've gathered insights from your friends and family, it's time to distill your brand into a captivating elevator pitch. This concise summary will be the foundation of your online profile. Think of it as a teaser that piques curiosity. It should highlight your unique qualities and create a desire to learn more. Avoid generic statements and set your sights on what sets you apart. Draw inspiration from successful brands that use concise and memorable messaging. Think Trader Joe's, not Val-Pak. Whether you're an avid reader, a travel enthusiast, or a community volunteer, there's a way to produce a compelling narrative that showcases your personality and interests. Your goal is to create an impression and spark connections.

Reach for your pen and get brainstorming!

WORKSHEET #5— YOUR ELEVATOR SPEECH

#11 Refine the Pitch to a Catchy Tagline

Condense the elevator pitch down to a tagline that summarizes you. Think of the successful brands you know. What makes them memorable? They have a clear, consistent message. Apply this concept to your profile. Develop a short, impactful tagline that summarizes your unique essence. Keep it concise, like the slogans of major companies. This tagline will be your personal branding statement in the dating world.
 So, here are a few examples to get your brain buzzing.

Solid Opening Lines: 10 Examples

1. Michael, 59, Brooklyn, NY.

If someone says, "Hey, would you like to_____?" I try to say "yes!" as often as I can. I have two Passports—one for International Travel and one for the National Parks—and I love getting both stamped.

Why do I like this one? Very quickly conveyed that he is adventurous without using that word.

2. Michelle, 66, Chicago, IL:

My favorite things:
- *Jeni's gooey butter cake ice cream*
- *A good fine pen and nice paper (I have over 200 pens—don't judge!)*
- *Annual Goodreads reading challenge*
- *Traveling (all 50 states and six continents —South Korea coming up this year)*

What do I like? It's great formatting and easy to read. Plus, men like women who eat! Michelle is a bit quirky about the 200 pens; it has elicited so many male responses. Men look at your photos first, and if you pass GO, they look at the first line or two of your profile. They just don't like to read, but Michelle made it easy for them.

3. Lauren, 53, Pasadena, CA:

I was raised on a horse ranch in Montana, but SoCal has been home for a long time. I was an athlete, from horseback riding and jumping to softball and skiing to cheerleading and hockey. I'm new to online dating.

What do I like? Few people who live in SoCal were raised on a horse ranch, so right away, it's different. Second, this client had never done online dating before, so it let people know how "new" she is to the app, which everyone online wonders about everyone else. (Why? If they've been on forever, maybe they are a "player" or not serious about a relationship and both men/women get excited when there's someone new!)

4. Angela, 62, Del Mar, CA:

Athletic and a Golfer for 40 years. (I've had two holes in one or is it two hole in ones?!?)

What do I like? The holes in one thing—men have been all over this—with comments about which it is. And, of course, she's a golfer, and so many men are interested.

5. Tim, 53, Atlanta, GA:

I am a recent transplant back to Atlanta from the San Francisco, CA, area. I am highly active, an award-winning artist, and an identical twin. My top priorities and loves are my twin daughters (24) and family. I am a Falcons season ticket holder—I hope you like football. I have taken so many cooking classes, and my friends say my Beef Bourguignon rocks. I hope you like to eat too!

What do I like? Tim just absorbed so much information so fast—just reading it, I got a love of family, football and food!

With that, what follows is **NOT** going to land great dates. Why? Yawn factor, big time. Boring and totally unoriginal. Hard pass. By the way, I didn't write these. **These are some I picked out online to help me fall asleep.**

6. Male, age 64, Boston:

"Love is not love
Which alters when it alteration finds,
Or bends with the remover to remove:
O no! it is an ever-fixed mark
That looks on tempests and is never shaken."
Shakespeare

Really?! This is not how to start your profile. Are we supposed to be impressed? This man went on to quote other people, too…and just that he loved these quotes, and we knew nothing about him.

7. Male, age 49, Dallas:

This is detailed for transparency (w/much more still unsaid) & I'm free to live anywhere! I am diverse, living by creeds like Carpe Diem & Joie de Vivre! Also, C.S. Lewis defines Agape as "a selfless love passionately committed to the well-being of another." So, I'm deeply focused & perceptive about my partner's emotions, needs & desires every day. My goal is to share a life of love, meaning, fun & happiness with a wonderful woman forever! True love combines romance, friendship, family & friends, and care for all humanity & nature. It's an all-encompassing physical, emotional, and spiritual sharing that defines every aspect of our lives, touching everyone we meet. As my favorite Bible verse says, "Without love, nothing else matters." I'm not a serial dater. I've had romances w/magazine models & other lovely, sweet, fun & interesting women.

Please, pass me the glass so I can eat it. Just stop. This is his formatting. Really, from the Bible to magazine models? And he wrote over 1500 words. He's full of himself and full of it in a non-appealing marketing way —red flag. Run.

8. Christoper, 60, Tampa, FL:

I am looking for my match and a long-term relationship, hopefully forever to. I work from home and can live anywhere—and can live anywhere—will happily relocate too where my match live, if desired. You're happiness is my priority. You can go from jeans to a litle blak dress.

63

Umm—generic, icky, typos...does not know basic grammar. Obviously didn't spell check. And do you think he's going to move? The red flag is on fire on this one. Don't just run, sprint.

9. Jim, 56, Washington, DC:

I am a well-educated (Rhodes scholar, Harvard, masters Columbia), artistic, active, romantic, industrious, articulate, funny and fun-loving guy. A one-year scholarship to write my doctoral dissertation in Sweden turned into 14 years there, but eventually, I wanted more sunshine and a warmer ocean! I have had a long, successful career dancing, teaching and choreographing dance for television, professional theater and others in Sweden (a little brag: I was one of the choreographers of the opening and closing ceremonies at the Summer Olympics in Tokyo in 2020)...

Humble braggart? Really? He came across as so wincingly impressed with himself that my client and I could not finish reading his profile. (Of course, I changed name, cities, IVY schools and venue of the dissertation). I'd bet significant bucks if you went out with his guy, you'd never have an opportunity to speak.

10. Cori, 68, Savannah, GA:

I'm enthusiastic, kind, active and creative. I was widowed 5 years ago—he was the love of my life. I'm not sure about online dating, as I know many weirdos and scammers are out there, but I was encouraged by a friend. I'm looking for someone to share an intimate, emotionally honest, long-term relationship with me.

Although I'm a homebody, occasionally I like to go to a nice lunch. I was a stay-at-home mom, and I enjoy taking care of others. Please only respond if marriage is your goal.

I read this one while working with a male client, and we both had the same reaction: We felt terrible for her, and my male client was turned off entirely too. Desperate and Debbie Downer. We both had the feeling she was not over her husband's death. Once again, to succeed in dating you must be ready—really ready.

#12 Cue the Makeover

Refresh Your Look for Dating Success

A makeover can be a powerful tool when re-entering the jurisdiction of dating. For women, updating your hair with a new cut or highlights can make a significant difference; or covering gray hair can help maintain a youthful appearance. Treat yourself to a facial and a complimentary makeover at the Chanel counter at Neiman's or Saks, and book in for that wax or hair removal session.

Elevate Your Self-Confidence

These steps not only refresh your look but also boost your self-confidence.

#13 Trim (or Better Yet) Shave that Beard

Why Grooming Matters: Creating a Polished First Impression

Many men have embraced the unshaven look in today's relaxed work environment. Yet when it comes to dating, a well-groomed, clean-cut appearance will always fare better and make you look younger. Nobody wants to see wispy gray hairs encircling your face. Just as a job interview requires a polished presentation, your first date is an opportunity to make a positive impression. A neatly trimmed beard or a clean-shaven face can enhance your overall appearance and project confidence.

Refine Your Hygiene Game: Grooming Tips for a Memorable First Date

I hate to break it to you, but nose hairs are a thing—especially as men exit their more youthful ears. If you can't do it yourself, ask around. Barbershops, medical spas and specialized grooming salons often provide such services. Don't be embarrassed. It's life. And it is a grooming hack that is well worth it.

First impressions matter, so take the time to refine your grooming routine. Extra effort can go a long way in creating a memorable first impression.

#14 Get Moving

Get Fit for Love:
The Importance of Physical Health in Dating

Let's be honest with ourselves here: nobody wants to be on a date with a special someone, struggling to reach the top of the stairs. Prioritize your physical health alongside emotional readiness. If you haven't already, consider joining a running club, diving into a team sport, hitting the gym, or investing in a personal trainer. Regular physical activity not only sculpts your body but also fortifies your mind.

How Exercise Boosts Mood and Confidence

Exercise is a proven stress reliever, boosting mood and confidence. It can help you feel more energized, positive, and attractive, translating into a healthier and happier dating experience. Physically caring for yourself is an investment in your overall well-being, enhancing your ability to connect authentically with others.

#15 Botox Filler Rules and Regulations

**Cosmetic Enhancements:
Timing and Tips for a Natural Look**

Considering cosmetic enhancements before diving back into the dating pool? Great! Timing is critical. Botox and fillers can work wonders, but rushing the process can lead to less-than-ideal results. For optimal outcomes and to avoid any potential bruising or swelling, schedule your appointments at least two weeks before your first date or photo shoot. This gives your skin ample time to recover, ensuring a natural and refreshed look.

Subtle is Key

When it comes to fillers, less is often more. Subtle enhancements are crucial to achieving a polished appearance without appearing overdone. The overdone, duck-lipped, puffy, I-just-stepped-off-a-Las Vegas-stage show look doesn't make you look younger or better. (This applies to men and women!)
If this is a route you want to take—and it is very individual—do your research, find a skilled injector, and allow enough time for the magic to work its way.

#16 Seek Out a Personal Shopper

Embracing a Fresh Look for Renewed Confidence

There's nothing quite like retail therapy and a fresh look to inspire a renewed sense of self-assuredness, making you feel ready to make a great first impression. You also want to dress your age. You can still be fashionable without needing to resort to the 25-year-old daisy dukes or the sleeveless summer shirt that rocked in your second year of college.

The Benefits of a Personal Shopper and Wardrobe Refresh

When preparing to re-enter the dating ocean, seeking out a personal shopper can make the world of difference. In other words, guys we don't want you to dress like your dad and gals same rule applies. We want you to be you—but the smart, sophisticated and absolute best part of you. Before I started dating, I decided to treat myself to a personal stylist. It was a fun and eye-opening experience! My stylist helped me try on clothes I never would have chosen, and she had a great sense of style that was both trendy and age appropriate. I learned a lot about how to update my wardrobe without looking too young or too old. Four new looks are a smart investment.

Personal shoppers at stores like Nordstrom offer free services to help you update your wardrobe. Inform them of your goal to find 3-4 new dating outfits that are crisp, casual, and modern. A personal shopper can also help you select new accessories like stylish Italian eyeglasses. These updates enhance your appearance and boost your confidence, ensuring you don't look outdated. Embrace this opportunity to refresh your look and feel your best. It's an investment in you, and in finding the right fit. No pun intended.

#17 Configure Your Color Scheme

The Power of Color Psychology in Your Dating Profile

Beyond the content of your profile, the visual elements play a crucial role in capturing attention. Keep this in mind when purchasing your few key clothing pieces. Just as businesses carefully select color palettes to evoke specific emotions, you can leverage color psychology to enhance your online dating presence. Imagine the impact of a bold, confident red profile picture versus a washed-out, forgettable one. Colors convey personality and can leave an impression. Incorporating strategic color choices into your profile can make you more memorable and appealing to potential matches.

You need to consider this before photo time, too.

**Preparing for Photos:
Choosing Colors That Reflect and Elevate You**

Want to be memorable? Consider why a First Lady often wears red—to stand out. You'll rarely see drab colors on the red carpet at the Met Ball. What you wear and the colors you choose speak volumes. For instance, red evokes passion and action, much like McDonald's and In-N-Out Burger's marketing. While designers may favor beige for interiors, they use vivid accents like orange or lime green to add vibrancy. Don't be afraid to be noticed; we want to play on the minds of those who come across our profile. Infuse your photos with bold colors to stand out.

While the color scheme you choose should not only reflect you but complement your coloring and complexion. Again, this is where the personal shopper at your department store works wonders!

#18 Pay Attention to "Down There"

**Balancing Comfort and Style:
Footwear Tips For First Dates**

Shoes speak volumes on a first date. They're a subtle yet powerful indicator of personal style, diligence, and overall presentation. Comfort is a cornerstone. However, flip-flops, Birkenstocks, and Crocs project a casualness that might not align with a first-date impression.

If you must go super casual, opt for a well-maintained pair of dress sneakers for a balance of comfort and style. A quality brand shoe, even a sneaker, conveys care and consideration.

The Devil—and God—Are in the Details

People notice details, and your footwear is a key component of your overall look. It's a small investment that can yield significant returns in how you're perceived.

#19 Tailor Those Clothes and Accessories

The Impact of a Tailored Wardrobe on Confidence

A well-tailored wardrobe is the cornerstone of a polished appearance and putting your best foot forward, with confidence to boot. Investing in alterations can transform even the most ordinary outfit. From hemming pants to adjusting shoulder seams, tailoring ensures that your clothes fit flawlessly, accentuating your body type and boosting your confidence.

**Accessorizing with Precision:
The Finishing Touches**

Beyond clothing, pay attention to accessories like glasses and jewelry. You want those to fit exactly right, too. Again, it's not just about the clothes you wear, but how they make you feel. A confident and stylish appearance can leave a lasting impression.

#20 Mani (and, Heck, Why Not the Pedi) Time

**The Importance of Well-Groomed Nails
for a Great First Impression**

Well-groomed nails make a positive impression on a first date. Men notice nails. Women do, too. They are an indicator of our hygiene and self-worth. We especially notice if they are dirty or not well maintained. Hence, a nice set of nails tells us that you take care of yourself and pay attention to the details. Bonus, a fresh manicure or pedicure can boost your confidence and make you feel more put together, thus oozing a calmer and more confident demeanor. People, add this to your to-dos.

#21 Whiten That Smile

The Power of a Bright Smile: Making a Lasting First Impression

A smile is one of the first things that grab attention. Those pearly whites (or not so white) can be a massive turn-on—or off. Whether you're a man or a woman, investing in teeth whitening can significantly enhance your appearance and boost your self-esteem. A bright, white smile conveys good oral hygiene, overall health, and a cheerful outlook. I tell all my clients, even those who think their teeth are fine, to make the effort. Consider whitening your teeth before re-entering the dating arena a non-negotiable. Even a slight improvement in teeth color can remarkably impact your overall look. So, don't hesitate to brighten your smile.

Investing in Teeth Whitening: A Must for Re-Entering the Dating World

Give your dentist a call today. Teeth whitening can be done in the chair in an hour or two, or the take-home kits also work wonderfully and tend to be much more budget friendly. Personally I like the med-spas—very reasonable and the same quality as at the dentist.

#22 Professional Photos Are a Must

Why High-Quality Photos Are Essential for Your Dating Profile

High-quality photos are incumbent for creating a compelling online dating profile. While relying on selfies or casual snapshots is tempting, professional photography can make a significant difference. (No, I'm not talking about that cringe-inducing, posed Golden Girls Glamour shots popularized in the 1980s). A skilled photographer can capture your best angles, use flattering lighting, and create images that reflect your personality. Avoid outdated studio-style photos and opt for natural, candid shots that showcase your lifestyle and interests. First impressions matter; your photos are often the first opportunity to connect with potential matches.

Tips for the Perfect Dating Profile Photo Shoot

An important tip: The magic hour for photos is undeniably the golden hour, that enchanting period shortly before sunset. Outdoor lighting during this time is simply unmatched, casting a flattering glow on everyone. That's why scheduling your photo session about an hour before twilight is ideal.

Your photos will be stunning, and you'll have the rest of the afternoon to relax and prepare for any evening plans. You may also want to consider getting your hair and makeup done professionally (hair first!), but emphasize that you want to look *like you*.

Reference #1

(See #42 for Guidelines for Online Profile Photos, detailing the photos you need and how to find the best pro!)

#23 Master the Art of Listening

A Little-Appreciated Key to Successful Dating

Effective communication is a cornerstone of any successful relationship. In the dating arena, being a good listener is vital. Start now. Get good at it before that first date arrives. Use every conversation you have as an opportunity to be present and improve your skills. Focus on actively engaging in conversations, showing genuine interest in the thoughts and feelings of those around you. Avoid interrupting and dominating the conversation. Instead, ask thoughtful questions and offer supportive responses. By demonstrating that you value the perspective of others, you create a deeper connection and build trust. Relationships are built on mutual understanding and respect.

#24 The Importance of Being Well-Read

**Expand Your Topics:
Engaging Conversations Beyond the Basics**

Aside from your career, kids, family, and golf game, have other engaging topics to discuss. Whether it's a recent film, a book you're reading, new restaurants you're exploring, or current events, discussing interesting things makes you more alluring. It doesn't matter if you read the *Wall Street Journal* online daily or prefer the New York Post; being informed and having diverse interests can spark great conversations and showcase your well-rounded personality. My go-to? For a quick daily news roundup, check out 1440. It's a free online resource that curates interesting articles in just a few minutes. It's a great way to stay informed without spending hours reading.

**Staying Informed:
The Key to Being a Great Conversationalist**

A well-rounded individual is an engaging conversationalist. Stay informed about current events, keep up with the news headlines of the day, take a little time now to delve into thought-provoking books, and explore diverse interests. Cultivate a curiosity for the world around you.

Whether discussing the latest film, sharing insights on a trending topic, or exploring a shared passion, being well-read opens doors to stimulating conversations. Knowledge is power, and it can be incredibly attractive in the realm of dating.

#25 Have a Social Media Presence

Curating Your Social Media Presence for Online Dating

Before you say it, nope you are not too old. Social media has become an extension of our identities in today's digital age. Before diving into online dating, curating a social media presence that accurately reflects who you are is crucial. A well-maintained profile can offer potential partners a glimpse into your professional and personal life and showcase the things in life you love. Further, you build trust and authenticity by showcasing your interests, values, and accomplishments. A robust online presence can be a powerful tool for connecting with like-minded individuals.

Key Platforms and Tips for an Impressive Online Presence

If you can only do one platform, make it LinkedIn and ensure your professional information and accomplishments are up-to-date and your profile picture is (again) recent and taken by a pro, bringing out the best in you. I also recommend Instagram, which doesn't require a huge amount of labor as you can throw up a few pictures—a careful curation of your life. (You can skip posting dancing videos on TikTok unless, of course, your moves are pretty darn impressive!)

On this note, if you already have social media now is the time to give it a detailed review and remove anything that doesn't propel you into the best light. Have your dating coach, or a trusted friend, also give it a once-over for any red flags.

#26 Be Mindful of Those Negative Nips

First Impressions Matter: Avoiding Negativity in Early Interactions

When interviewing potential employees for It's Just Lunch, I typically began with benign questions: "Did you find this place okay?" or "How was parking?" If they responded with complaints, the alarm bells immediately shrieked in my head, telling me all I needed to know about that potential hire. Needless to say, they didn't get the job.

The same applies to dating, just as in business interviews, where a negative attitude towards minor inconveniences can be a dealbreaker. Early dates are when people usually try to present their best selves, so it will be a massive turn-off if someone is already churning out the negatives.

Nipping Negativity in the Bud: Being Mindful of Your Attitude

The moral of the story? Don't let that person be you. Be mindful of when you are complaining, when the glass is half empty, and what you can do to nip that negativity in the bud. We don't want you to drag that into the dating field. It just isn't cute.

#27 Ditch the One-Track Type

Most of us dive into the dating pool with preconceived ideas of what exactly we are looking for, and in the process, we let potentially amazing prospects drown. Let's wretch open that mind, shall we?

Breaking Free from Preconceived Notions in Dating

Spare me a moment to tell you about one of my former clients, 47-year-old Amy. Amy was a force of nature, a whirlwind of creativity and ambition that swirled through the heart of New York City's fashion scene. Her designs were bold, edgy, and undeniably her own, a reflection of the city's relentless energy.

Yet, for all her success in the cutthroat fashion world, Amy's personal life was different. She had a type: tall, dark, and driven, the quintessential Wall Street power player. But despite their shared ambition, these relationships always ended in disappointment. The constant pressure to perform and be the perfect partner to these high-powered men left Amy feeling drained and unfulfilled.

Slowly, a realization dawned on her. Her search for a partner was as misguided as the trends she once dismissed. True compatibility lay outside the narrow confines of her preconceived notions. With a newfound openness, Amy began exploring connections beyond her usual circle. She discovered that intelligence, humor, and shared passions were far more attractive than a seven-figure salary or a handsome exterior. And so, the fashion icon, once obsessed with finding her perfect match, embraced the adventure of discovering love in unexpected places.

Yes, she found love with a classic nerdy type in science years ago, and they couldn't be happier.

**Keeping an Open Mind:
Real-Life Lessons in Finding Love**

Rigidly adhering to a specific "type" can significantly limit your dating options and potentially hinder your chances of finding a truly compatible partner. By keeping an open mind, you expand your horizons and allow yourself to discover unexpected connections. Everyone has unique qualities and experiences that contribute to who they are, and focusing solely on superficial attributes can overshadow deeper compatibility.

Women often tell me repeatedly on weekly coaching calls as we are perusing potential dates online, "Oh, no, Andrea, not him. I've seen him online for 5 years." Okay, you wait! (Big parenthesis… you've been online looking for 5 years yourself before becoming my client with no success—yet you won't reach out to a man in similar straits?) As I said, wait!

To give you a little more hope on the open mind front, I'll tell you about one of my clients, Lara, a spunky, funny, athletic, and attractive 58-year-old from Palm Beach, Florida. We were looking through men online together (by phone) recently, and by the fourth time I've picked a high-potential date for her, she says the same thing for the fourth time, "No, I've seen him online for the past six years. He's a player."

Okay, I'm direct. Very direct but graciously direct as my only interest is you ending up in my 65% success column of clients who are in long-term relationships.

Me: "Lara, and you know he's a player how? And you've been online how long?"

Lara: "That's different. I'm picky."

Me: "I bet he is too. I read his profile. He seems lovely. I want you to give him a try, and by next week when we have our coaching call, I can't wait to hear about your date."

Reluctantly, she did. Reached out. Date scheduled. Turns out to be an interesting and kind man. He'd been traveling quite a bit with work and getting three kids settled in colleges and internships as a single dad the last four years with not much time to look at his online dating app. He told Lara he was grateful she'd reached out. Fingers crossed Date 2 goes as well.

#28 Nobody Wants to Be on Dating Apps Forever

Understanding the End Game: Insights from Real Clients

Of course, there is an end game to all this. And the more we know, the more strategic we can be with our time. To arm you with a little more information, I am sharing an interview with two of my male clients on what they are seeking. No, they are not identical—just as no two of my clients are alike! What they had in common was that they wanted results and didn't want to spend much time messaging women online. One commented he'd rather be on the golf course than on a dating app; the other has an intense career and plays basketball in his free time—neither of the men's idea of fun was online dating. Surprise, surprise, right?

Stay tuned for dating advice they have for women near the end.

Behind the Profiles: What Men Really Want and Their Dating Advice

Here are the facts: Mark, 64, a business executive from Dallas who traveled 85% of the time, had serious time constraints. Tim, 55, Silicon Valley, technopreneur and founder who lived primarily in New York City.

Why Did You Decide on Online Dating?

Mark: *I realized I wasn't going to meet anyone where I worked where I worked---it was highly discouraged, plus I was a high-ranking executive at a Fortune 100. I was divorced for 5 years. I had two teens at home, and I was just ready to date (not a serious relationship, I thought). I knew nothing about online dating, but I had seen commercials.*
Tim: *These days, I haven't seen any other choice. Everyone is doing it! I looked at the company you founded, Andrea, It's Just Lunch, and couldn't imagine they had a large enough pool compared to the internet. When I researched the numbers on the online dating pool, it seemed an easy decision.*

What Were Your Feelings about Going Online?

Mark: *Hesitant. I fear people recognizing me (and it happened twice—a woman from my neighborhood who I actually went on a date with and a woman from my company whom I did not date). At this point, I got over my fear of people recognizing me. I thought, hey, our senior VP of Marketing is online, so I got over it!).*
Tim: *My hesitation was privacy---people will see you unless you choose the option where they only see you if you select them, but then you are limiting your choices. Another drawback was time---not to get caught up looking at these damn sites all day long---well, that was until I hired you, and you wouldn't let me. (He laughs).*

How Long Were
You on the Sites/Apps before Hiring Andrea?

Mark: *5 years. I just had no time and would check it once a month, which, of course, was not optimizing my dating life. I went on 4-5 dates a year but wasn't putting much effort in. Then my kids went off to college, and I hired you and got more serious. I didn't even know someone like you —a dating coach—existed five years ago. Hey, I was married for a long time!*

Tim: *I was married for 24 years and initially got lucky online and was in a relationship for 9 months. I then went on 3 sites/apps for three months, which was overwhelming. That's when I decided I needed help and hired you to vet these women and show me a more efficient way to use online dating.*

How Often Did You
Check the Dating Site/App?

Mark: *Once a month.*

Tim: *Every day before you. I'm super organized and tend to check emails constantly, too, but I quickly got swamped with the dating thing and became discouraged/frustrated with time and energy.*

What Three Things Make a Woman Attractive and Make You Want to Reach Out? And How Did You Respond? Message, Phone, or Straight to a Meetup?

Mark: *Her photos and something in her profile made me laugh, or we had a commonality (like one woman who was also from Boston, where I grew up and visited the Cape as often as I do)—a message on the app, then a text, then a short phone call. I did the phone because I'm a bit reticent and shy, so hearing their voice first made the in-real-life meet feel more comfortable and like a second date.*

Tim: *All the things you preach! Multiple photos, a complete profile, and listing things that are unique to them---no generic platitudes. As far as the first date, I think women want to feel safe, so I'd take the lead from them—I'd say 50% we just agreed via text to meet at a restaurant, and the other 50% we had a short phone call after a couple of texts. It just depended on them.*

Have You Ever Thought about Using a Matchmaker or Doing Group Single Events?

Mark: *Definitely not my style at all. I wasn't comfortable with either of those.*

Tim: *No. In today's world, it makes no sense. Do you really need a "travel agent" these days, or can you book your own hotel and flights? Now, having someone write your profile, select photos, set me up online and help choose dates—that's cost-effective.*

What about Your Photos?

Mark: *I initially picked a couple- one with family and friends- to show I was social. Full body. A few women told me men misled on height (I'm 6'2), so I ensured there was a full body shot, too. And I was smiling. You had me add more—no baseball cap and only one with shades on!*

Tim: *Typically, 5. Headshot, activity (at a football game or concert), hiking. I wanted to show my entire body in shorts and a T-shirt.*

What Advice Would You Give Women Online Dating?

Mark: *Stand out by saying unique or quirky things about you. I liked this one woman who was funny and quirky and said "I have two sets of twins in their late teens, no I can't tell the girls apart which can cause mayhem, I just mastered my pasta machine and pesto recipes with anything green I can find including broccoli and I've won three competitions this year with my favorite bow and arrow.*

Tim: *I frankly got mad when I met someone where it was obvious that they were using old photos. My advice to women is always to date your photos.*

Anything Else We Should Know?

Mark: *Hire someone like you. It saves time, and you'll be on the right track.*
Tim: *My dog photo got a lot of comments! So did the one playing pickleball with my 15-year-old, though I covered her face. It's just showing the real you.*

Thanks, Mark and Tim. Okay, so you want to know their outcome. Mark's in a committed relationship—as he told me early on, never say you'd never marry again! Meanwhile, Tim has been with Gail for a year; they don't live together nor plan marriage—but it's a committed relationship.

Here Comes the Flipside:
What Are the 11 Things Women Want Here?

Having worked with thousands of women over the years and listened to countless date stories and anecdotes, I've found some commonalities in what women look for in a partner.

1. Equality: Whether you're 30 or 60, women today value independence and seek partnerships in relationships. The man is no longer the sole "hunter." Think about your best friend relationships with your girlfriends - they're based on equality, right? Romantic relationships are no different.

2. Chemistry: Without chemistry, it's just a friendship. Attraction is key, and it may not be instant on the first date. It often develops by Date #3 or 4. Ever been on a first date where someone seemed average-looking, but by the end, their conversation and mannerisms made them more attractive?

3. Stability: This includes financial, emotional, and relational stability. Someone who shows anger issues or gets upset easily is not emotionally stable. We're all on our best behavior initially. If you see any red flags regarding stability, move on.

4. Curiosity: This means being curious about you and wanting to get to know you. It also means being curious about the cosmos around him, having interests, and being open to trying new things. Relationships need to grow, and that can't happen with someone lacking this trait.

5. Assertiveness: This doesn't mean being bossy or controlling. It means knowing what you want in life, a relationship, and the future. Women appreciate this trait as well - that's what makes a partnership. Ever dated someone who constantly defers to you for decisions? It gets frustrating and boring quickly.

6. Encouragement: This goes both ways. Maybe you're considering a career change, a trip, or a course. A good partner listens actively and supports your endeavors.

7. Sexual Satisfaction: Our needs may change from our 20s, but an active and fulfilling sex life keeps the spark alive in a relationship. Intimacy is critical.

8. Surprises: Who doesn't love a thoughtful gesture? It can be a loving note or flowers for no reason. Grand gestures aren't necessary - it's about showing you care.

9. Keeps Promises: He follows through on his commitments. Whether it's a call, weekend plans, helping you, or watching your pet - he's dependable. These little things show he's trustworthy.

10. Trust: The example of Angie (a client in her 60s) highlights the importance of trust. Her date's jealousy and phone-checking behavior were red flags. There are plenty of good men out there - don't settle for someone who makes you question his trustworthiness.

11. Age Preferences: Many women believe men only want to date younger women. This is a misconception. Statistics show that 80% of men prefer to date women around their own age. So, don't worry about the minority who seek younger partners. Let them do their thing, there are plenty of more appropriate options for you.

#29 Commit to an All-in Effort for at Least 6 Months

The Emotional Rollercoaster of Online Dating: Don't Give Up

Online dating can be an emotional rollercoaster, often leading to premature discouragement. It's common to feel disheartened after a few unsuccessful dates, tempting many to give up after three weeks. But don't do it! Don't give in! While a rare few may experience success right off the bat, it takes at least three weeks for the magic to start to materialize. Online dating isn't a crazy quick fix. Remind yourself, you've come too far to quit now. We're just getting started.

**Perseverance Pays Off:
The Key to Success in Online Dating**

Perseverance is core in navigating the online dating sphere. Just like building a successful business or mastering a new skill, finding love requires dedication and patience. While the initial weeks may involve trial and error, it's during this time that promising connections can begin to form. By committing to at least three months, you increase your chances of encountering someone special. Countless people have found lasting love through online platforms, proving that persistence and an open mind are fundamental.

The color **ORANGE** encourages enthusiasm and adventure in **Navigating the Digital Landscape.** Approach online dating with curiosity and openness.

chapter 4
Navigating the Digital Landscape

#30 *Diversify Your Dating Portfolio*

Successful businesses don't rely solely on one marketing channel. They employ a multi-pronged approach, combining advertising, public relations, and word-of-mouth. While I'm not suggesting these exact tactics for your dating life, the principle holds true: cast a wide net. Instead of limiting yourself to a single platform, create profiles on two or three popular dating sites and/or apps. Dedicate three months to fully immersing yourself in these platforms.

Dating Apps and Sites—What's the Difference? Let's Break It Down

- An app that is typically used on a mobile device cannot be accessed on your laptop, while a dating site is primarily used on a laptop or desktop, but often has an accompanying app.

- Dating sites tend to offer better search functionality on a laptop. To maximize your efficiency, avoid using your mobile for this purpose. For example, when working with clients over 50 who primarily use dating sites, I insist on using a laptop.

- I've even recommended that clients purchase an inexpensive laptop for this purpose. Your time is valuable, so don't be cheap if you're serious about finding success.

- Apps provide less information and rely heavily on photos. Your photos must be exceptional to stand out.

- Because app bios and prompts are limited, your responses need to be unique and engaging. Consider hiring a professional dating writer for both apps and sites.

- In all honesty, both sexes struggle with writing dating profiles and dating prompts. Women tend to be too long and unfocused; men tend to be short, terse or try to skip this completely. Both may benefit from a female dating coach as both men and women find speaking to a woman easier.

Which Is Better?

Is one better than the other? While more people over 50 use sites, there are exceptions. Apps tend to appeal to a younger demographic, but they are gaining wider acceptance with the over 50 crowd. A multi-tiered approach can offer diverse opportunities and get your profile into various parts of the population. The sites below are inclusive to all dating preferences!

#31 Platforms to Go for

Let me get a little more specific on the sites I like for the 45/50/60 plus crowd.

6 Reasons Why You Might Want to Use an Over-50 Dating Site

1. Focused Age Group: You'll be matched with people in your age range, avoiding unwanted attention from much younger users.

2. Reduced Gold Digging: These sites tend to attract users seeking serious relationships, minimizing encounters with those motivated by financial gain.

3. User-Friendly Interface: Designed for Gen X and Baby Boomers, the interface is easier to navigate than platforms aimed at younger demographics.

4. Long-Term Relationship Focus: Many over-50 sites cater specifically to users seeking long-term commitments.

5. Enhanced Safety Features: They may offer more robust security and privacy settings, giving you greater peace of mind.

6. Local Activities: Some sites organize group events for users in your area, providing opportunities to connect outside the online realm (especially in major cities).

**Maybe Not for Everyone:
2 Considerations for Over-50 Sites**

1. Subscription Costs: These platforms often require paid memberships, which may be a drawback if you're just browsing.

2. Limited User Base: Depending on your location, the user base might be smaller than on broader dating sites.

**Analysis of Top Sites/Apps:
Experience Speaks Volumes**

Some of my advice comes from research, however, it's heavily influenced by working with over 35,000 clients online. I've witnessed firsthand which platforms work best for specific goals. Online dating trends constantly evolve, so what was effective in 2005 is no longer a fit for 2025.

**Match.com:
My Rating YAY (Site and App)**

1. Pros: Match.com is the oldest dating site and is primarily a platform for those seeking serious relationships. It reminds me of shopping at Target; you see every type of car in the parking lot, from Mercedes to beat-up Corollas. Similarly, Match caters to a diverse range of people, from young to old, and from highly educated to vocational backgrounds. The Match Group owns a dozen other dating sites and apps (at least 45 at the time of this writing). As the second largest dating site among over 1400 worldwide, Match offers an unparalleled user interface and search functionality. The platform requires a detailed written profile, which must be well-fashioned to attract potential matches.

2. How it Works: you can search for other members, send messages, and arrange dates. All communication happens within the site, including phone calls and video chats, providing an extra layer of safety for those who prefer not to share their personal phone number initially.

3. Cons: Given the platform's vast size, finding compatible matches can be challenging if you lack a clear strategy. To avoid unexpected charges, it's essential to note your cancellation date, as all dating sites and apps typically bill your credit card one day before the subscription ends. Avoid purchasing add-ons such as boosts and matchmaker services; I have found these to not work.

4. Tip For Success: Fill out EVERYTHING on this site. It will take you an hour if done right. This will increase your ranking.

5. To Pay or Not to Pay: ALWAYS PAY. I recommend the 3-month Premium Membership.

6. Final Tip: Only reach out to Paid Subscriber. No one else. If they aren't willing to put a little coin in the game, they aren't really serious.

Bumble: My Rating YAY (App)

1. Pros: Women make the first move, which empowers them to initiate conversations with men. The user base tends to be more educated overall. The app includes a good photo verification feature, so users can be confident that they are interacting with genuine profiles.

2. How it Works: Download the Bumble app on your phone or iPad from the App Store or Google Play Store.

3. Profile Setup: Creating a profile is easy. Upload your photos, write a brief bio, answer a few questions, and select your preferences. Matching is done through a swipe system

4. WOMEN: As a woman, you must be proactive in liking profiles and starting conversations. If you don't take the initiative, no interaction will occur.

- **Cons:** You might exhaust your potential matches in your area. To avoid frustration after the initial influx of matches, check the app less frequently after the first two weeks. The location tracker can be problematic, especially if you travel. For example, if you live in Chicago but travel to San Diego, your Bumble feed will primarily show San Diego-based users. The app lacks a search function, and user availability may be limited outside of major metropolitan areas.

- **Tips:** Turn off this App when traveling. This app's benefits are contingent on user engagement. Bumble has a hidden ranking system that determines your visibility. This ranking is influenced by how actively you interact with the app, such as liking profiles, responding to prompts, and engaging in conversations. While many users are unaware of this system, it significantly impacts your experience.

- **How to Connect:** You have a 24-hour window to send a message after matching with someone. If you don't initiate contact within this period, the match expires. This system helps keep your inbox manageable.

5. MEN: Since women take the first step, you might enjoy not having the constant pressure to initiate contact. This app is user-friendly for men, as there's often a good pool of potential matches available. You have 24 hours to respond to a message. Bumble's straightforward design makes it easy to navigate. To increase your visibility, respond to messages promptly.

Our Time: My Rating YAY (Site and App)

OurTime is owned by the Match Group and shares many of the same features. The site offers a terrific search engine that allows you to easily filter potential matches based on various criteria. OurTime specifically targets the over-50 age group.

The platform is user-friendly and easy to set up but allocate about an hour to complete your profile thoroughly for optimal results.

1. Pro: OurTime provides good customer support, frequently asked questions, and helpful blog articles.

2. Tip: Always purchase the 3-month premium membership for the best experience.

3. Pro: The site offers strong safety features, including profile verification.

4. Con: OurTime may have a limited user base in certain areas.

5. Tip: Consider using OurTime in conjunction with a different platform that utilizes a personality-based matching system, such as SilverSingles. I recommend using two dating sites for the over-50 demographic: a universal platform like Match and a more age-specific site like OurTime. The only issue you may notice is the overlap of the same people between Match and Our Time as often daters use both.

6. Tip: When using two dating sites, devote your attention to one platform for approximately two weeks to familiarize yourself with its features before adding a second site.

(Note: If on a budget, choose Match.com over Our Time, as there is much overlap.)

#32 Platforms to Avoid

There are apps and dating websites to avoid, even some of the big names. It is not necessarily because they don't work, but more because you don't get much bang for your buck, they just don't have the pull and aren't right for the 45 to 65 demographic.

Hinge: My Rating NAY (App)

Owned by the Match Group, Hinge utilizes detailed profiles and prompts. It is primarily used by a younger demographic, aged 20-45, and is exclusively available as a mobile app.

1. Tips: Use the rose feature to express strong interest in a profile and stand out from other users. Be specific when responding to prompts or asking questions, focusing on information shared in the user's profile. Hinge's algorithm tracks user engagement with profiles.

2. Cons: Hinge has a limited user base within the over-50 age group and has minimal safety features.

3. Pros: Potentially suitable for individuals in their 50s seeking partners in their 30s or early 40s.

JDate: My Rating NAY (Site and App)

Traditionally catered to Jewish singles seeking matches, the platform that has declined in popularity.

1. Cons: Limited user base and an outdated interface, with a search-based platform.

Many former JDate users have transitioned to more mainstream dating sites like Match, OurTime, and Bumble.

Raya: My Rating NAY (App)

Raya has positioned itself as the "Tinder for Celebrities." Its membership is invite-only, and gaining access is often seen as a status symbol. The app vets potential members based on factors such as industry and social media presence.

1. Pro: Raya can be beneficial for networking purposes.

2. Cons: Extremely expensive (costs thousands of dollars), primarily caters to a young demographic (20-45, with a heavy emphasis on 20s and 30s), and is irrelevant outside of major metropolitan areas like New York City and Los Angeles. Additionally, the acceptance rate is low, leading to high frustration levels for many applicants.

Oh, and contrary to widespread belief, Ben Affleck was never a member of Raya. I've had clients receive invitations to Raya, and I don't think it is all what it is cracked up to be. Be warned if that invite does surface in your inbox, you are going to see more twenty-something artists and hipsters in far-flung parts of the country, and even the globe, than you will see the Tom Brady's and Brad Pitt's of the world. In other words, it isn't worth your time or money.

Sites I Absolutely Do NOT Recommend.

1. Christian Mingle (Site and App): Offers a small user base for the price and suffers from outdated technology and frequent glitches. You'll have better results using common dating sites with Christian filters.

2. Badoo (Site and App): While categorized as a dating app, Badoo also functions as a social networking platform with a global user base. It's notorious for fake profiles and scams.

3. Ashley Madison (Site and App): This site facilitates extramarital affairs, which contradicts the goal of finding a committed relationship. It's known for fake profiles, undesirable users, and a history of data breaches.

4. Microsites (such as): Clients often suggest these niche sites, but I strongly advise against them. It's preferable to find suitable matches on more reputable platforms. In reality, these microsites are typically low-quality, overwhelming users with spam, and a waste of time.

- Liberal Hearts (for Democrats)

- Conservative Dates (for Republicans)

- Environmental Dating Sites

- Yoga and Meditation Dating Sites (a complete waste of time; consider attending a yoga class or an ashram retreat instead for a more authentic experience)

- Seeking and other "Millionaire" sites

#33 Some "Maybe" Platforms to Consider

EliteSingles: My Rating MAYBE (Site and App)

A dating site targeting educated professionals, which employs a personality testing methodology for matchmaking.

1. Pros: EliteSingles verifies user profiles.

2. Cons: Both the platform and membership are expensive, and the user pool is small. The site's user interface is not particularly user-friendly, and matches may be located across the country. It had its day and the numbers here have seriously declined.

Results vary widely. Some clients have found success on EliteSingles, while others have had negative experiences. The platform's effectiveness is heavily dependent on location, with rural and suburban users reporting less success.

The League: My Rating MAYBE (App)

Originally designed for graduates of Ivy League and similar institutions, The League has expanded its eligibility criteria to include a wider range of universities. Once accepted, users receive suggested matches, although the quality of these matches can vary.

1. Pros: Targeting ambitious professionals, The League verifies users through their LinkedIn and Facebook profiles. Potential members must complete an application and join a waitlist before gaining access. Despite claims of long waitlists, acceptance often occurs quickly.

2. Cons: The platform is expensive, offers a limited number of daily matches, and can be frustrating for users in less populated areas.

Users can pay extra to increase their daily match count.

eHarmony: My Rating MAYBE (Site and App)

Well-known for its in-depth compatibility matching system based on extensive questionnaires, eHarmony is historically recognized for facilitating long-term relationships and marriages.

1. Pros: Strong safety features, numerous success stories (although many are from over a decade ago), and performs well in smaller markets.

2. Cons: The sign-up process is lengthy, users often disregard their personality test results after initial enthusiasm, and there's limited control over suggested matches. From its inception, this site has not kept up with easy user interfaces and also a very limited client base in many markets.

Tinder: My Rating MAYBE (App)

Tinder is the largest dating platform globally, including the United States. It offers a simple, swipe-based interface.

1. Pros: Tinder is easy to set up. Add photos, write a brief profile, specify age range and location, and begin browsing. It also performs well in both large and small markets.

2. Tips: High-quality photos are a must-have for success. Be sure to clearly define your relationship goals, whether it's a long-term partnership or marriage. In recent years, Tinder has introduced premium features to attract an older demographic and emphasize serious relationships. A paid subscription is highly recommended. While Tinder Select is very expensive (approx. $499/month), there are better options like Tinder Gold and Tinder Platinum coming in at under $30/month.

I've successfully used Tinder with some clients over 50, but it's not ideal as a first-time online dating experience due to its overwhelming nature. Be explicit about your relationship goals, focusing on long-term partnerships rather than casual encounters. The platform moves quickly, so users must adapt to its demanding environment. A premium subscription is strongly advised.

That is barely the tip of the iceberg. There are thousands upon thousands of niche websites from Coffee Meet Bagel to ones that accept only high credit scores, to ones for the unvaccinated and others that align to your political views. I could go on and on. As a rule of thumb—my words of wisdom—stick to the well-run power players mentioned above. Wasting time in the weeds of these smaller ones will only frustrate you, not to mention drive you mad seeing the same face show up several times a day given the limited number of users in the niche market.

Facebook Dating: My Rating (MAYBE)

1. Pros: Facebook Dating is easy to use, with a simple interface and integration with existing social media. It has strong geographic targeting, which is effective matching based on location preferences. In addition, FB Dating has a wide user base, making it suitable for both urban and rural areas, especially for the over-50 demographic. Another bonus? Its privacy control feature—the ability to hide your profile from Facebook friends.

2. Cons: There is the lack of commitment. This is a free platform that often attracts users seeking casual interactions rather than serious relationships. There are also concerns over profile quality; many users have inactive or poorly maintained Facebook profiles. Finally, it can be a limited pool with the potential for running out of matches in smaller communities.

#34 Pay to Play

Maximizing Your Dating App Experience: Are Premium Subscriptions Worth It?

While not every premium feature on dating apps is worth the cost, and these can run into the hundreds of dollars every month, investing in a basic subscription can significantly enhance your experience. Platforms like Match benefit from a three-month premium membership, unlocking game-changing tools to expand your search.

Focusing on Core Features: Getting the Most Out of Your Subscription

Tinder, for instance, has evolved into a more relationship-focused platform, particularly for the over-35 demographic, making a paid subscription worthwhile. To truly maximize your chances on apps like Hinge and Bumble, a premium membership is often necessary. (But this doesn't mean you need to purchase all the bells and whistles on offer!)
While additional bells and whistles might tempt you, homing in on core features can provide a solid return on investment.

#35 Engage, Engage

The Three-Week Mark: When Dating Apps Start Working in Your Favor

I promise you things will start to improve after three weeks if your initial experience hasn't been ideal. This isn't just encouragement; it's based on data. Dating app algorithms are designed to keep users engaged and maximize platform usage. To achieve this, the apps often prioritize active users. Increased visibility typically occurs after the initial three-week period as the algorithm assesses your commitment. Consistent engagement, such as liking, commenting, and frequent app use, signals to the algorithm that you're an active user. What the algorithm really loves is more than just a passive like, but a two-way interaction. Write a response or respond back to a comment from someone else. Do it daily. Multiple times a day.

Daily Engagement Tips: Maximizing Your Reach and Match Quality

This increased activity expands your reach and enhances the quality of matches as the app learns your preferences. Prepare to put in the hard yards. This doesn't need to feel like a chore but can be an incredibly fun daily investment that will—if you stick it out—deliver the goods.

#36 Farewell the Common Misconceptions

Oh yes, many people have them. So, let's dive right in and dispel the three I hear the most…

"No Way Will I Like Him"

Let me share what happened recently — and I know my client in the Southwest is reading this. Cari is a new client, as we were reviewing potential matches for her online, she kept saying, "No way."

I have a 50/50 rule when choosing dates. To simplify the decision-making process for dates, I use a 1-100 scale. A 1 means 'absolutely no way,' while a 100 indicates 'ready to pick out a wedding dress.' While the 'no's' are usually obvious, many potential dates fall in the 50-80 range, making it more challenging to decide. If you are more than a 50 out of 100 on going—go.

In Cari's case, I was getting exhausted with her excuses, so I chose three men and told her I was going to write them an initial message on the dating site we were on together. (She exclaimed, "No, they should reach out to me!" My reply: Why should the men do all the work?) Women making the first move is hot, and it doesn't mean that chivalry is dead.

On a follow-up coaching call, Cari told me about her 4-hour date with John on Saturday—how they laughed, how much they had in common (and didn't—that's the spice of life!), and how much better he was in real life. This is the man she did NOT want to meet. They have another date this weekend, so we'll see what happens. Well, at least I didn't say, "I told you so" because I was so happy!

"Listen to Your Friends"

Back to Cari again. She was resistant to the site we were using because her "friends" didn't like it. Translation: They met no one because they didn't know what they were doing. Her friends were negative... and single. Once I told her I had three engagements on this site alone in one month, she was a bit pacified. Please, listen to an expert dating coach with experience, not friends and family.

"If They're Attractive and Successful, They Wouldn't Need a Dating Site"

Paradoxical, right? You're here, aren't you? And so, is Matt, a successful 54-year-old Upper East Side Manhattan doctor, widowed with two teens still at home—exactly where is your love life supposed to sprout from? Your practice? I think not. Friends' one-off dates? Nope. I'm reminded of my client Carl from a year ago in Nashville in the exact same situation.

He told me to get to work; he just wanted to date. He trusted me and let me do my job, just like I'd trust him in the ER. A month ago, I got a text from him, on a glacier in Switzerland with his fiancée, Mira. Yep, they met online.

#37 Avoid Early Blustering and Burnout

The First Few Weeks of Online Dating

Let's talk about how to avoid getting burned out in the first few weeks. If you recall, in my experience, I signed up for way too many sites at once, losing myself in the early vortex. By day 10, I was sending messages like crazy, excited about the possibilities. However, by day 16, I was a total mess! Five first dates in a week left me exhausted and confused. I couldn't remember what I said to whom. That's why keeping a dating log is imperative.

Below is your dating log, which requires just a little input before and after your dates. Trust me, a few minutes of your time will save you a big headache and maximize your chances of success.

Navigating the Digital Landscape

Building a Sustainable Routine: The Power of 21 Days

But again, here's why 21 days are key: It takes time to develop a rhythm. The first 10-12 days are about building a routine. Aim for 2-3 sites, spending 30 minutes a day building those quirky messages. By week 3, you'll be a pro—messages flow naturally, like chatting with someone you already met at a cocktail party last week.

Just a side note that I will reiterate multiple times throughout this book: Don't fall into the "oneitis" trap. Just because you had a great third date doesn't mean you should ditch those other promising first dates. Keep exploring options until you're in an exclusive relationship. Schedule no more than two first dates per week. This allows you to manage your social energy and avoid burning out.

Even though I always pushed myself to the brink a couple of weeks in and got so sick of it, I did follow my own advice and push past the 21-day discomfort, reminding myself that I, too, committed to at least three months. I started in May and on July 21—between that illustrious two-and-three-month mark—I met Jeff, who would become my husband.

Andrea McGinty

WORKSHEET #6—
Dating Log

When **Crafting the Perfect Profile,** the color **AMBER** symbolizing warmth and approachability. A well-crafted profile should feel genuine and welcoming to potential partners.

chapter 5
Crafting the Perfect Profile

#38 Keep It Short, Sweet, and Quirky

Balancing Brevity and Authenticity

Crafting an effective dating profile requires a balance of brevity and authenticity. Short, engaging bullet points are preferable to lengthy paragraphs. Highlighting unique qualities is a must-do but avoid bragging. We want you to keep it honest and concise, with an emphasis on your interests and versatility. Nobody wants a one-dimensional partner who just goes to the gym, or just works, or just talks about sporting teams.

Crafting the Perfect Profile

**Show, Don't Tell:
Creating a Standout Profile with Personality**

For public figures, downplaying high-profile occupations can deter unwanted attention, while simultaneously conveying your passion for the special things in life. To create a stop-in-your-tracks profile, focus on showcasing your personality through vivid examples rather than simply stating facts.

5 Tips for Writing Your Profile

1. Focus on your personality: What makes you unique? What are your interests and hobbies? Use humor if it suits you.

2. Be specific: Instead of saying "I love to travel," mention a few favorite destinations or travel experiences.

3. Use strong action verbs: Words like "explore," "create," or "adventure" can make your profile more dynamic.

4. Show your values: What matters to you in life? This can be a great conversation starter.

5. Proofread carefully: Typos and grammatical errors can create a negative impression.

Example Profile Structure

1. Headline: Short and intriguing (e.g., "Adventure seeker with a soft spot for dogs")

2. Photo: A clear, recent photo of you smiling.

3. Bio: Short bullet points highlighting your key personality traits, interests, and what you're looking for in a partner.

#39 Ask a Question

Make Your Profile a Conversation Starter

A finely tuned dating profile should be more than just a list of your interests. It should be a conversation starter. One effective way to achieve this is by asking engaging questions. Instead of simply mentioning your love for travel, why not ask, "What's your dream travel spot? I'd love to hear about it." This not only shares your interest but also invites potential matches to share their experiences, sparking a connection.

Crafting the Perfect Profile

Engagement is Key:
The Power of Personal Touches

I often receive unsolicited pitches from businesses eager to revamp my social media or website. Generic, overly critical emails are quickly deleted. However, personalized video presentations with thoughtful feedback and engaging questions have a much higher chance of capturing my attention. This approach mirrors the effectiveness of a good dating profile: genuine interest and an invitation to interact.

#40 Throw in a Super Bowl if You Desire

Stand Out with a Unique Conversation Starter

We want to give all the suitors out there the perfect opportunity to contact you. One trick? Include a mention of your favorite Super Bowl commercial on your profile.

For me, Super Bowl Sunday is more about the commercials than the game. Think about your favorite ad and let it be your springboard. Not only does it highlight your personality, but it also gives potential matches an effortless way to start a fun and engaging conversation. After reviewing countless dating profiles, I've realized that humor is an often-overlooked superpower.

#41 Target Your Niche. Know Your Niche.

Appeal: Crafting Profiles with Purpose

La Creuset advertising on the Food Network is targeting foodies, not the Monday night football crowd. The Golf Channel is not running ads for Tampax. For example, as a male seeking a woman online, you are not seeking quantity, only quality. So broad sweeping statements like "walks on the beach and can wear a tuxedo as well as jeans" are just stupid, meaningless, and boring. We can do better.

WORKSHEET #7—
CRAFTING YOUR DATING PROFILE

Crafting the Perfect Profile

#42 Choosing the Best Photos

Making Your First Impression Count

Ah, the most important component of your dating profile is, for better or for worse, your photographs. We live in a visual society, and that is just that. There is no escape from it. Your photos are your first impression, so make them count! Ditch the boring selfies and LinkedIn headshots. Show off your fun side with action shots that capture your interests. Think golfing, hiking, or even juggling (yes, really!). People love to see someone who's enthusiastic about something. Take note, a photo of you volunteering or hanging out with friends says way more about you than a stern-faced headshot.

Keep it real, keep it fun, and let your photos tell your story!

Andrea McGinty

Let Your Photos Tell Your Story: Guidelines for Success

Below are the guidelines that I share with all my clients with proven tips and tricks on the photography front. Don't forget, a personal dating expert is also an invaluable resource in helping you select the best snaps!
Some sites/apps will allow only 5 photos, some up to 25! It is especially important to choose photos that represent you! Not oldies but goodies! They say a picture is worth a thousand words (or something like that!), and it is never truer than with online dating!

1. The magic number is 6-8 photos to post.

2. When you are sending them to me for review, please send me up to 20 so we can cull the photos.

3. I strongly recommend that you hire a professional photographer! It will make the world of difference. You can have a strong bio, but if your photos are subpar they will be passed right over, we do live in a visual universe. Please see my tips below for hiring a pro and making it a huge, high priority as we go through the online dating process together!

4. All photos should be taken in the last 12 months.

Crafting the Perfect Profile

5. Photos should include:

- One fun headshot smiling (not a corporate photo—this is your love life not resume!)

- At least one full body shot: this can be you hiking, doing an activity, standing in front of your Christmas tree, holiday-oriented photo.

- A shot playing with your pet is always fun. Dogs are much more popular than cats

- No sunglasses. Everyone likes to see your eyes!

- Keep a photo with a hat on to one maximum

- Travel photos are fun, but you must be in the picture too!

- 1-2 group photos are fine. Maybe it's you and your children, a group of friends at a wine tasting, sailing, etc.

- Playful photos are fun and show off your personality!

- Outdoor shots are great with colorful backgrounds: mountains, water, gardens, ruins, but again, you need to be in the photo

- Shirts on! (I am talking to you, guys!) Exception would be if you are water skiing, etc.

- Photos of you with your interests: tennis, golf, yoga, traveling, pickleball

- No selfies unless you have one (just one) that is fantastic

- Smiling!

- High resolution 1MB, no grainy or blurred shots

- If you wear glasses, include a few photos minus your glasses

- Stiff photos will not work—posting 6-8 photos where you are directly smiling at the camera will look phony and contrived---If you are using a professional photographer, make sure they know this. So, in-studio photos typically won't work
- Ski/cycling shots. Take your helmet off for the shot if possible

9 Tips for Women

1. If you are going to have some professional photos taken (which I highly recommend), tell the photographer that you are using these for your online dating profile.

Crafting the Perfect Profile

2. Most clients tell me this has cost them between $250-$500.

3. Have the photographer take both indoor and outdoor shots

4. Hit the hair salon that morning. You will look great with a fresh blow-out!

5. Good dental care matters—it may be time to stop by the dentist to have your teeth cleaned and whitened. Do this one week in advance.

6. Bring some props, your furry friend, a golf club, a racket, and a Santa hat. This is your license to be creative.

7. Before the photo shoot, speak to the photographer about anything you can bring to "fun" up the photos and let your personality shine.

8. Bring 5-6 changes of clothing: from a dress to athletic wear to jeans and casual attire.

9. Bring extra jewelry. We don't want these shots to look as if they were all taken on the same day! How about eating an ice cream cone? Yep, men like women who eat….and it's a cute photo!

13 Tips for Men

1. Action shots. You are engaged in a sport or activity you like

2. Walking your dog (or your mom's, sister's, etc.)

3. Eating a favorite food. It could be a loaded pizza or a slice of watermelon (these types of photos are real!)

4. Again, hire a pro!

5. 5 different shirts (jeans/shorts)

6. Gardening, backyard shot

7. Swimming Pool shot

8. Boat shot

9. No photos in your car or by your car unless you have a serious car hobby

10. No selfies in the mirror

11. If you can have a friend take some outdoor full-body shots, great! (throwing a snowball with a baseball jersey/bat, or tennis racket; those work well)

12. Shave! Clean cut sells better.

13. Whiten your teeth—there are many places that will do this in an hour. Your smile and teeth… really matter!

Free Printable Form

Psst… want my expert photo shot list, along with a cheat sheet to hand to your photographer? Head to **33000Dates.com** *for your free, printable form.*

WORKSHEET #8— PHOTO FORM QUESTIONS/CHECKLIST

#43 Show not Tell

Okay, so let's talk about showing off your formidable qualities. It's nice to say you're a family person, but actions speak louder than words, right? Social media is a wonderful place to share real-life stories about your life. Tell everyone about hosting a huge holiday dinner for your whole family. That's way more interesting than just stating you love family time. But what tops that? Show us a picture. Show don't tell.

**Show, Don't Tell:
Highlighting Your Life Through Photos**

I had one 60-year-old client who wanted to express his family-oriented side. How did he do that? He used a picture with his 90-year-old mother on St. Patrick's Day, kissing her forehead. It was adorable. Another client, a grandmother, used a picture of herself dressed identically to her five grandchildren in matching Hanna Andersson pajamas with the Christmas tree twinkling behind them. That, too, spoke volumes.

Prioritize your family and have a penchant for the outdoors? Another client killed two birds with one stone—posting a snap of him and his three sons hiking Mount Rainier. People really connect with this approach. It's like, "Wow, this person is actually the real deal!" Not just someone who says they are.

Crafting the Perfect Profile

Let Your Photos Speak: Capturing the Essence of You

Before asking a question, as I mentioned earlier, it is all about showing, not telling, too. Love to surf? You could show a cool pic or ask, "Bondi Beach or the North Shore?" on the prompts. A wine lover? "Château Margaux or Robert Mondavi?"

Again, 6 photos should tell your story. Even if the site allows for more than that, don't do it. Sum it up in 6.

#44 The Low-Down on Featuring Others

Strategic Group Photos: Showcasing Your Social Side

Using photos with other people in your online dating profile is acceptable and can showcase your social proclivities. If you post a group shot, ensure you are front and center, and there is no confusion over whose profile it is. A group photo should never be the first image a fellow user sees. Blurring or emoji-covering the faces of others is not necessary; more than likely, your friends or loved ones couldn't care less, except in the case of young children, say fifteen or younger.

#45 Inject Humor into Your Profile

Make Your Light-hearted Self Stand Out

Humor is a powerful tool for connecting with others. Incorporate wit and charm into your online dating profile to stand out from the crowd. A well-placed joke or a playful anecdote can make your profile more engaging and memorable. Don't be afraid to showcase your personality and let your sense of humor shine through. A little self-deprecating humor can be disarming and attractive. By injecting laughter into your profile, you'll increase your chances of finding someone who shares your sense of fun.

Unsure where your sense of humor lies? I can help!

We all think we have a good sense of humor. Clients often tell me they do, emphasizing that past dates lacked humor. But wait... could it be *you* who lacks humor?

Crafting the Perfect Profile

Understanding Your Humor Style: A Key to Connection

This "sense of humor" thing has been prevalent for over 3 decades in my career (yes, I roll my eyes). It's because, well, I *am* funny (just kidding... mostly).

Back in the 90s, when I started It's Just Lunch (pre-33000Dates.com), clients listed three desired characteristics. "Sense of humor" was always on the list, alongside "kind," "active," "adventurous," or "serious about a relationship." Some even claimed to laugh all day at life's trivial things, never getting down (excuse my skepticism here).

Vanilla. (That's why I avoid vanilla ice cream. There is no surprise or spunk in it.)

These words are meaningless. Used in online dating profiles, they get you nowhere (except putting readers to sleep), just like they do to me while coaching clients and reviewing bios/prompts.

Now, back to humor. There are so many types: dry, silly, self-deprecating, witty, weird, Monty Python-esque... or the classic, "I have a great sense of humor if it's funny to me."

Here are some different, albeit common types of humor to think about:

15 Humor Types Based on Delivery and Style

1. Slapstick: Physical comedy involving exaggerated actions and often silly or clumsy behavior.

2. Deadpan: Humor delivered with a serious, expressionless demeanor.

3. Wit: Intelligent and quick humor, often involving wordplay or clever observations.

4. Sarcasm: A sharp, often ironic or satirical form of humor.

5. Dry humor: Understated, subtle humor that relies on irony and unexpectedness.

6. Black humor: Humor that deals with dark or taboo subjects.

Crafting the Perfect Profile

Based on Content

7. Observational humor: Humor based on everyday life situations and observations.

8. Self-deprecating humor: Humor that makes fun of oneself.

9. Satire: Humor that uses irony or wit to criticize society or individuals.

10. Absurd humor: Humor based on illogical or nonsensical situations.

11. Dark humor: Humor that deals with serious or taboo subjects in a humorous way.

Based on Personality

12. Affiliative humor: Humor is used to build social bonds and connect with others.

13. Aggressive humor: Humor used to put others down or gain a sense of superiority.

14. Self-enhancing humor: Humor used to cope with stress and maintain a positive outlook.

15. Self-defeating humor: Humor used to deflect attention from oneself or to appear humble.

Andrea McGinty

Most people exhibit a combination of these styles, and humor can vary depending on the situation and audience. Have some fun today and put a name on your humor. Here are some fun quizzes that may help you define your level of humor; or surprise you.

Have at it:

- https://www.quizexpo.com/what-is-your-sense-of-humor/1/
- https://www.buzzfeed.com/hazelyxlee/comedies-good-sense-of-humor-quiz
- https://www.buzzfeed.com/eliachuaqui/eat-some-crazy-desserts-to-determine-your-true-sen-cwlrlpic9x
- https://quizly.co/what-is-your-sense-of-humor-percentage/

A Little Exercise

After you describe your sense of humor on a dating site (if you have one, sorry, some people just don't so move on to your other amazing qualities) then ask what sort of sense of humor do you have? You could even include one of the links above. Brilliant conversation starter if I do say so myself!

#46 The Want-Kids-Someday Prompt

One thing that can be a bit of a turn-off on dating apps is when you see a man, especially one over the age of 55, who has marked "Wants kids someday" on his profile. I've seen this quite a bit, and it often makes me think, "Why would they select that or do they really?"

The Confusing 'Wants Kids' Checkbox: What It Really Means

Half of my clients are male, so I often review their online profiles. When I ask them why they chose that option, they usually respond with something like, "I don't actually want any more kids, but I'm trying to keep my options open—just in case I meet a woman in her early 40s who hasn't had children yet."

It's the sort of prompt that comes with a double-edged sword. Women often tell me, "I don't want to go out with him because he's open to having more children, and I'm 50—I'm not having any more kids." But my advice is usually, "Who cares? Go out with him. You're not marrying him on a first date! Everything else about him seems great. You've already messaged and connected well. If the topic of kids comes up, you'll find out that maybe he doesn't actually want more—he just didn't fill out that part correctly.

**Decoding Profile Prompts:
Focus on the Bigger Picture**

It's a reminder that sometimes people select certain options on their profiles without fully thinking them through. It's similar to the "420 friendly" prompt. If you're anti-marijuana and someone is consuming it multiple times a day, that's one thing. If it's not a deal-breaker, there's no need to stress over it. Some things just aren't worth worrying about. The kid prompt doesn't need to determine if you go on a first date or not.

#47 Be Careful of Cliches

**Avoiding the Usual Photo Pitfalls:
Why Your Gym and Selfie Shots
Aren't Helping**

I love that you love the gym, your bathroom, your seatbelt and travel—but we need to be careful to evade the cliches when putting that out there. In other words, jettison the sleeveless shirt (or worse, no shirt) gym pic. Yuck. The same goes for the bathroom mirror selfie and the selfie of you in your car. Just no. And on the travel front, and I don't mean to sound too brutal here, but tourist trap pictures in places a generous portion of the country have been to aren't going to cut it. Translation: say no to the photograph of you throwing a coin into the Trevi foundation or standing at a bazaar in Istanbul.

If you want to showcase your zest for travel, do so only if the picture is especially unique and cool—riding a camel at sunset in Jordan's Wadi Rum desert, trekking through the Amazon rainforest, or making handicrafts in a tiny Lebanese village. That is interesting, and that is the question to ask yourself: does this photo stand out? Is it a conversation starter? Is it really that interesting?

Highlighting True Adventure: The Difference Between Real and Cliché

The same unspoken rule applies to conveying a sense of adventure. Are you a qualified solo skydiver? Amazing. I would love to see that. Are you doing a tandem jump? Good for you, and I applaud your bravery, but it is not for your dating profile. If adventure is truly your thing, the photo should be a jaw-dropper for it to work: I'm talking about summiting K2 Mountain or kayaking in the Arctic. Those definitely aren't cliches.

Car Enthusiast or Poser?
The Right Way to Showcase Your Love for Cars

The car thing? If you really love cars down to the bone, or maybe you're a car collector, a photo in front of a Ferrari would work in conjunction with a little explanation about your love for the sport or vintage collections. But going to Miami and posing beside someone's cool McLaren on Ocean Drive? Please, no.

Rethinking the Fishing Photo:
How to Make It Stand Out

The same question marks swirl around the guy holding up a fish photo. Every one of my female clients will tell me how often they see this, and almost everyone will roll their eyes. If you must post a fishing photo, let's make it a little different. A beautiful location at sunset, a still ocean, and a contemplative moment are far more alluring than the tried-and-true dude holding up his whatever.

Showcasing Your Workout Wisely:
Flattering and Fun Choices

If you like working out, that is fine to showcase—let's be strategic about it. For example, a yoga picture can work wonderfully, but let's skip the unflattering downward dog. Warrior or tree pose is great, or if you are carrying a little more weight, a seated lotus or half-lotus is flattering. Or if Pilates is your jam, add some levity to it—doing a plank on the reformer with your puppy right beneath your face? That is cute. What I am encouraging here is to think outside the box.

Unique Talents in the Spotlight: How to Make Your Hobbies Shine

What else is interesting? Showcasing a talent. Especially if it is a talent off-the-beaten track. I had one client who is a buttoned-up, super serious, Wall Street guy. But the picture that landed him immense success in the digital dating cosmos was the one of him at a street fair in Brooklyn juggling pomegranates. Sometimes, pictures (the right ones) catch our eyes and speak a thousand words.

#48 Putting Your Politics Out There with Caution

Treading Lightly for Better Connections

This is a cautionary light. While it's tempting to flaunt your political affiliations on a dating app, especially if you feel very strongly one way or another, it's often wiser to exercise restraint. Briefly mentioning your political leanings in one of the bio prompts that most apps allow you to do is fine, yet I would advise against waving partisan flags in your photos or wearing shirts that explicitly pin your politics. Dating apps are about connection, not political rallies. Save them for Facebook or Instagram.

Keeping It Neutral:
Why Excessive Political Expression Can Backfire

Excessive political expression can alienate potential matches and create a divisive atmosphere. Focus on showcasing your personality and interests, and let your political views emerge naturally in conversation if the opportunity arises. In addition, writing statements such as "if you supported XYZ then don't bother swiping right, followed by a rant…" is a waste of valuable dating profile space and doesn't frame you in an attractive light.

#49 Seek Feedback from Friends

Getting the Right Input:
Why Selective Feedback Matters

Seek feedback, but wisely. As a solid rule of thumb, I recommend showing your profile to three people. At least one should be a member of a different sex, such as a sibling, your best friend's spouse, or a close colleague who knows you well and also knows their gender pretty well. This diverse feedback will give you a well-rounded perspective on your profile.
  I had one gorgeous client who had really stunning professional photographs taken. What I didn't know after we selected the photos and built the profiles was that she then went and put those photographs through major self-editing—so much so that she looked like an AI cartoon.

Crafting the Perfect Profile

"I would never ask you out if I saw those photos; they are so overdone that they don't even look real," her brother exclaimed.

Thankfully, she listened to him and reverted the photos.

Avoiding Overkill:
The Pitfall of Too Many Opinions

Getting input on your dating profile can be valuable, but avoid oversharing, as too many opinions can cloud your confidence. Too many cooks... you know the drill.

#50 Update Your Profile Regularly

Profile Refresh Strategy:
Stay Visible and Intriguing

Keeping your dating profile fresh and engaging is vital for attracting potential matches. Regularly updating your profile at least once a month helps you stay visible and interesting. Rotate your primary photo to maintain intrigue, and remember that quality trumps quantity when it comes to images. Six carefully selected photos are often more effective than a larger, less focused selection.

**Engaging Updates:
Fine-Tune Your Text for Better Results**

Don't be afraid to experiment with your profile text. Adjust prompts that aren't generating interest and replace them with more engaging questions. For instance, instead of simply stating, "I love scuba diving," ask, "The Great Barrier Reef or the Galapagos Islands?" This sparks conversation and reveals shared interests.

#51 Bypass the Scammers

Online dating can be a fantastic way to meet someone special, yet it's vital to stay vigilant against scammers. Here are some alarm bells to watch for:

5 Critical Alarm Bells

1. Be extra cautious on free dating apps without verification. Paid platforms, or those without stringent verification requirements, often attract individuals more serious about relationships. Scammers are more prevalent on free sites where they can create multiple fake profiles without financial investment.

2. Beware of Limited Photo Profiles. A profile with only one image is suspicious. Legitimate users typically include multiple photos to showcase their personality and interests.

Crafting the Perfect Profile

3. Delayed In-Person Meetings. Constant excuses to postpone meeting in person could indicate a scammer's reluctance to reveal their true identity. The FBI's website offers valuable resources on this topic.

4. Excessive Personal Questions. Be cautious if someone asks for an unusual amount of personal information early in the conversation. This could be data-gathering for potential identity theft or other malicious purposes.

5. Poor Grammar and Spelling. While not always indicative of a scam, frequent errors can suggest a bot-driven fake profile, or someone whose native language is different than claimed.

#52 The Two-week Travel Dating Rule Two

Dating While Traveling: Should You Give It a Go?

Another important topic: dating while traveling. Dating apps like Tinder and Bumble will recalibrate based on your geographical location. So, should you go on dates if you're visiting a different city, or is it better not to bother?

The key consideration here is how movable you are. If you're someone who can live anywhere in the country—which I'd say applies to about half of my clients—then yes, you can definitely date while traveling.

But there's a catch. No one wants to date someone who's only in town for three days. You need to commit to being in that city for at least two weeks before going on a date that is worth yours, and the other person's time and energy.

For example, I have a client, Adrian, who lives in Sun Valley, Idaho. He is completely movable, so I identified three good markets for him to date in: Denver, Seattle, and Santa Barbara —places Adrian likes and can easily move to. I told him he needed to plan to stay in one of these cities for two weeks at a time (though a month is better if you can swing it). As Adrian works remotely, he can work from any location, but the point is to be there long enough to make some real connections.

Setting Yourself Up for Success: Preparation Is Key

If you're going to try this, you need to plan ahead. Start prepping your profile about two weeks before you arrive. Change your location to one where you already live rather than say you might move there. If your profile says you're currently in Sun Valley, people may not take you seriously. If it says you're in Seattle or Santa Barbara, and you're genuinely considering moving there, you'll have a much better chance of making meaningful connections.

So yes, you can absolutely go on a date while traveling, but do it the right way. Commit to spending enough time in the city and preparing your profile accordingly.

#53 Looking for Tea and Red Flags? Not So Fast

The Risks of Joining "Are We Dating the Same Guy?" Groups

"Are we dating the same guy?" groups are online (mostly Facebook) communities where individuals can share information about potential partners they've met on dating apps or websites. There are counter "Are we dating the same girl?" groups. However, they have much less reach and relevance. In any case, these groups often use specific jargon, such as "looking for tea" (information) and "red flags" when someone wants to warn others about a date or an ex. While these groups can provide a sense of camaraderie and support, I strongly advise against posting photos of your dates or joining these groups beforehand. Doing so can create unnecessary drama, damage trust, and, overall, just plant an unnecessary seed of negativity in your brain. (Additionally, avoid linking your social media accounts to dating apps, as some may request access to your personal information, which can be invasive. Another point I will drill down!)

Avoiding Unwanted Drama: Think Before You Post

Moreover, if you have a bad date, take a long, hard think before you post that person's image and information under the "red flag" umbrella. Was he or she just rude and obnoxious, or are they a serious safety threat? Or just not your type, and you are disappointed? Or he didn't ask you out again? That does not make him a bad person.

Dating is hard enough without adding layers of drama to the mix. In short? Stay away from the "exposé" groups and use the time you may spend commenting and scrolling toward the much more effective goal of finding your special somebody.

#54 Outside the Online Dating Sphere.

While much of this book concentrates on digital dating and navigating the sites and apps space (it really just is the way to do it these days!), there are other options you may want to consider—including more traditional matchmaking.

Beyond Digital Dating: Exploring Traditional Matchmaking

The dating industry, particularly when it comes to matchmaking, can sometimes feel a bit like the used car sales business—it darn sure has a seedy side. You'll find people who are just out to make a quick buck, especially among those who offer "exclusive matchmaking" services. These matchmakers can charge anywhere from $50,000 to $200,000. I've referred clients to such services before, but I'm very selective about what ones are worthwhile and suitable for certain clients, only referring three or four a year.

Understanding Services Like Talkify and It's Just Lunch

You may have also seen ads popping up for the likes of Talkify and wondered what it's all about. (I'm sure the internet algorithms are—at this point—sending you all sorts of tailored dating-esque ads!) Let me explain. Talkify, along with services like It's Just Lunch, operates as matchmaking services/dating services within their own specific pools. They don't go outside their established member base to find matches.

For example, in a market like Washington, DC, Talkify or It's Just Lunch might have around 300 members. So, when they're matching you, they're selecting from that limited group. These services are not cheap, ranging from $6,000 to $7,000 for membership, though occasionally, a client might snag a deal for less. They usually guarantee around six dates.

Tiered Breakdown of Matchmaking Services

Now, if we're talking about tiers of dating services beyond online dating, here's how I would break it down:

1. Online Dating: This is the easiest and most accessible option. It's the lowest barrier to entry, but it comes with its own set of pros and cons.

2. Mid-Tier Matchmaking Services: This includes services like Talkify and It's Just Lunch. They operate within a confined pool of members in specific cities. The cost can be significant, but they offer a more personalized experience than online dating.

3. Local Mom and Pop Matchmakers: These matchmakers operate in specific markets like Charlotte or Orlando. They've usually been around for 10-20 years and have built a small, loyal client base. They charge around $10,000 for their services, but they only work with a limited pool of people within that area. Sometimes, they also host singles events, though these can be a bit of a hit-or-miss. You will find many of these only work with men and won't work with women over the age of 50. It's just not their forte.

4. High-End Matchmaking: This is where you can see the real success stories. These matchmakers charge between $50,000 and $250,000, but their methods are thorough. For example, I had a client in Laguna Beach who worked with one of these high-end matchmakers. The matchmaker didn't just rely on her existing pool; she actively scouted potential matches across Southern California, reaching out to connections on LinkedIn and beyond. This level of dedication often results in success—my client ended up engaged by the end of it. The matchmaker had an over 90% success rate, but you do pay a premium for that kind of service.

Understanding Traditional Mindsets

It is also important to address the traditional mindset that men should be the ones paying for matchmaking. In today's world, I believe women should also be financially invested in the process. When both parties have skin in the game, the chances of success improve.

Other dating avenues like meetups and speed dating are also worthy of mention. These might seem like lower-tier options, but they're worth considering. Many clients who use high-end matchmakers also engage in these activities to increase their chances of finding the right person. The key is to diversify your approach—combine online dating with matchmaking or other in-person events to cover all your bases.

Let's go a bit deeper.

From Exclusive (Read "Expensive") to Budget-Friendly

- Note 1: If you're serious about finding a partner—whatever that looks like for you (living together, not living together, travel partners, twice-a-week theater and dinner companions, marriage, or an exclusive relationship)—you need to try at least three different approaches. The idea is to "throw it all at the wall and see what sticks."

- Note 2. Dating now is a lot different than in your 20s and 30s when marriage and having kids were the main goals. Thankfully, that's not something we have to worry about anymore!

1. Exclusive Matchmaking Services

- **Overview:** You pay for an experienced matchmaker to search extensively for potential partners, similar to how an executive recruiter would work.

- **Target Audience:** Relationship or marriage-minded individuals.

- **How It Works:** They don't just match you from a pool of paying clients; they conduct outreach beyond their existing network.

Crafting the Perfect Profile

- **Caution:** Most matchmakers in this category aren't worth the investment.

- **Andrea's Experience:** After 30 years in this business, I know almost everyone in the matchmaking industry. There are only 2-3 firms in the U.S. I would recommend, and a heck of a lot more I would not.

- **Challenges:** Finding these top firms is difficult since two of them don't advertise and operate more like exclusive real estate "pocket listings."

- **Pros:** High success rate, personal touch, very efficient.

- **Cons:** Costs range from $30K (low-end) to $250K, with most services in the $75K-$100K range.

- **Andrea's Tip:** You can't take your money with you. If you're serious about meeting someone, this option offers the best odds.

2. Local and "Mom-and-Pop" Matchmaking Services

- **Overview:** Every city has one. Usually run by a single person.

- **How It Works:** They mostly match within their small pool of clients (typically under 75). Results vary, and there are no guarantees.

- **Payment Models:** Often, men pay while women don't, leading to older men (50-60+) seeking much younger, attractive women. Some services flip this, with women paying and men getting free memberships.

- **Pros:** The matchmaker does the work for you.

- **Cons:** Limited candidate pool, costs range from $8K-$20K.

- **Andrea's Tip:** Ask if all candidates are paid clients—this improves your odds. Also, check the male-to-female ratio, as these services often lean heavily on female clients. Make sure they commit to a guaranteed number of dates within your stated preferences.

3. National Dating and Matchmaking Services

- **Examples:** *It's Just Lunch* and *Tawkify*

- **Disclaimer:** I founded *It's Just Lunch* in 1990, ran it for over 15 years, and sold it over 10 years ago. I have no current affiliation.

- **How It Works:** Both services work with a larger local pool through a central corporate office, typically with several hundred members in larger markets. They match within this pool and may offer more expensive personalized searches.

- **Typical Offers:** Usually guarantee a certain number of dates (e.g., 6 dates over 6 months or 12 dates over 12 months).

- **Pricing:** Highly negotiable; both men and women pay.

- **Pros:** Available in large and small cities.

- **Cons:** Reputation and success vary depending on who runs the local office.

- **Andrea's Tip:** Men, negotiate hard on pricing due to market imbalances. Women, insist on a guaranteed number of in-person dates, not just dates presented to you that you're uninterested in.

4. Dating Experts/Consultants

- **Overview:** Typically, industry veterans with 15+ years of experience. They guide you to the best matchmakers, dating services, or apps.

- **Cost:** $300-$500 per hour, with a minimum of 3-4 sessions.

- **Pros:** Saves time and provides industry knowledge to help you get the results you want.

- **Cons:** Success depends on the consultant's experience, industry contacts, and expertise.

- **Andrea's Tip:** When committing to a package, ensure you understand the timeframe and exact services. This should be clearly outlined in writing or on their website.

5. Dating Coaches

- **Overview:** Coaches assist with everything from profile writing, photo selection, and dating site/app recommendations to messaging strategies.

- **Additional Services:** Some also provide advice on wardrobe, conversation skills, and building confidence after a long relationship or marriage.

- **Experience:** Look for someone with at least 15 years in the industry, with a proven history, success rate, and testimonials.

- **Pros:** With over 1,400 dating sites/apps, a coach can help you get a confident start and stand out online.

- **Cons:** Anyone can call themselves a dating coach, so research their background carefully.

- **Andrea's Tip:** Know exactly what you're paying for and the timing of the services. This should be clearly stated in writing or on their website. Always talk to multiple coaches by phone (10-15 minutes) to find a good fit.

Crafting the Perfect Profile

- Watch my video at **33000Dates.com** on 9 questions to ask before hiring a dating coach.

6. Speed Dating

- **How It Works:** A two-hour event where you meet a new person every 3 minutes.

- **Event Structure:** Kept at a 50/50 ratio of men to women, usually focused on a specific age group.

- **Improved Over Time:** Modern speed dating events have better gender balance and age targeting.

- **Pros:** You'll meet at least 10 people in one night, and these events are available in every city.

- **Cons:.** Some find 3 minutes too short and stressful.

- **Andrea's Tip:** Go with no expectations, smile, and follow up with a coffee date if someone seems like they're in the "ballpark."

7. Meetups

- **Overview:** A relaxed way to meet new people while doing activities you genuinely enjoy or have always wanted to try.

- **Popular Groups:** Book clubs, hiking, dancing, music, trivia nights.

- **Pros:** Low-pressure environment, many people are just looking for friends, which makes it easier to connect.

- **Cons:** The primary concentration is social, not dating. Also, primarily women attend.

- **Andrea's Tip:** Choose an activity you genuinely enjoy, not just what you think will attract men or women. This is also a clever way to "practice" social skills if they've gotten rusty after a long relationship or old friendships.

Crafting the Perfect Profile

If a relationship is truly your goal, you'll need to be a bit adventurous and invest some time. Trying multiple avenues leads to the highest success. Let's get you out of your friend rut and routines with these ideas:

1. Take a Group Pickleball Clinic: The fastest-growing sport in the U.S., it's easy to learn and highly social. I made new friends and even got après-pickleball dates when I moved to the East Coast last year!

2. Dog Parks: Pet owners tend to be super friendly and easy to strike up conversations with.

3. Take an Adult Learning Class: From language courses to design workshops, these classes feed your brain while introducing you to new people.

4. Trivia Nights: Go with just one friend (no more), and you'll get paired with others. You'll have a fun time and avoid the awkwardness of striking up conversations at a bar.

5. Volunteer at a Shelter: Whether it's for the homeless or for animals, volunteering is a fantastic way to meet like-minded singles.

6. Try Speed Dating Again: Keep it fun and light!

7. Yoga and Pilates: Guys, this is your chance! The majority of participants are women, and it's great for your mind and body.

Other Ideas

Attend alumni events, join a new gym, or join a book club at your local bookstore.

The more energy you put into the dating domain, the more you'll get back. Clients often say, "Suddenly, my calendar is booked," not just with online dates but with quality singles from other levels of society.

Bright and cheerful, **YELLOW** signifies optimism. **The Art of the First Date** highlights keeping things light and positive to make the first date enjoyable and memorable.

chapter 6
The Art of the First Date

#55 Setting Expectations

First dates can feel overwhelming. I've been there. I get it. What is the best way to set expectations? To have none, zilch, zero.

**Setting Expectations:
Embrace the Neutral Mindset**

The trick here is to go into the first date neutral: think the date probably isn't going to be a meeting of the minds with your long-awaited soulmate, but it isn't going to be awful, either. There is no pressure; it is just one date. It's a fun opportunity to meet someone new. That's it. The question you need to ask yourself after the first date isn't whether you want to marry this person but whether you want to go on a second date. That's it. Nothing more.

The Art of the First Date

#56 To Call or Not to Call

No Pre-Date Calls: Protecting the Magic

If you live within a 30-mile radius of your prospective date, there is no need for a phone call before the date. I have found in my experience with clients that this can ruin the magic (or set preconceived notions) before you can connect with the other. Sparks don't fly on the phone. They fly when eyes lock, and we engage in conversation.

For example, I had one client named Leah, a 55-year-old stylist in Austin who matched with a guy in her zip code online. A few days later, they spoke for an hour on the phone and then texted furiously in the days before the date. (Another no-no—once the date is scheduled, there is no more back-and-forth aside from a quick confirmation text on the day the date is scheduled.)

Leah was convinced this was her next husband and told me, her girlfriends, her sisters, and her close colleagues he was the one. As you can imagine, the expectations were pretty high. Not surprisingly, it was painfully apparent that there was zilch chemistry on the first date, and Leah felt incredibly crushed and defeated as she had to tend to the questions from everyone shrieking, "Well, how was it? When is the big day?" Worse, it took Leah quite a chunk of time after that to mentally pull herself up and back into the game.

When a Call Makes Sense: The Distance Factor

So, no call. The only caveat to this rule is if you live outside that 30-mile radius. I have one client, Natalia, who lives in a rural area in central Virginia and has had to travel to larger cities or even neighboring states to date. In that case, a call is warranted before making the trek.

But on that note, I am not a fan of long-distance relationships unless one already intends to move to that place for personal or professional reasons. There are too many variables; while some work out, that is the exception, not the rule.

Ending the Call: Keep It Direct

So, what if you do a call for 10 minutes? How do you close it? I just see too much of people "chickening out" and saying, "Let's talk again." OMG. Why? No, no, and no. If there is a chance you'd like to see this person in real life, say this: "It's been fun chatting. Where would you like to go from here?" Ok, there will be one of two answers:

1. "Let's talk again tomorrow." No. How about this: "Oh, I'm not much of a phone talker and like meeting in person. I'm free Thursday and Saturday for lunch. Does that work?"

OR

The Art of the First Date

2. "Let's meet." Great. Exactly what we want to hear. Have in your Rolodex a few ideas of meeting places so you are not stammering and hemming and hawing for a place to meet.

When I did my first dates, I kept it simple. I met all my dates for lunch at Deck 84 in Delray Beach, FL--- and it was funny as the hostess knew after a while and would say, "Oh, Andrea—he's out on the deck". It was my comfort spot!
Dating closer to home is a far wiser approach with greater odds of success.

#57 Give a "Which Day Works?"

The Invitation: Make It Count

You've exchanged a few messages, and it's clear you have things in common. The conversation has been fun and engaging. Then, one person sends, "We should get together sometime." What? That comes across as minimal interest or a lack of confidence. You know what sometimes means? Never!

The Art of the Ask

How about this instead: "Let's definitely get together this week—does Saturday lunch or late Sunday afternoon drinks work for you?" It's specific, shows genuine interest, and makes it clear that you're making time to meet. And importantly, it's not in the distant future! Online dating moves quickly, so there's no need to hesitate. This message says, "I'm confident you'd like to meet me."

By the way, this approach works for all sides—gone are the days when only the man does the asking.

#58 Managing Nerves

Overcoming Initial Nerves: The Power of 3

Know that those nerves, which can sometimes be pretty intense, won't last forever. When re-entering the dating whirlpool, the magic number is 3. Once you have 3 first dates with 3 different people under your belt, something just happens—the walls go down, your confidence grows, the conversation flows (no rhyme intended), and things just start to click.

Keep Your Circle Small: Avoid Pre-Date Discussions

I would also advise abstaining from discussing the date with your friends beforehand. We love our single pals, but I see too often that they have nothing positive to say about the process, and our committed friends in long-term marriages or relationships just aren't going to be on your wavelength with this one. So, keep it close to the chest.

#59 Choosing the Right Time and Place

Avoid Monday Dates: Choose the Right Timing

First up, don't do dates on a Monday. Why? Monday's are stressful for most people in the working world, with too much on the mind. However, Monday evenings are great for hopping online and engaging with the apps!

Skip the Coffee Date: Opt for a Relaxed Atmosphere

Second, I don't recommend coffee dates, even those at cute hipster coffee shops. They are just too informal and lack the ambiance for a first impression. I'll be frank: alcohol works. It just does. Instead of coffee, a relaxed atmosphere, like a happy hour at a nice bar, allows for better conversation and a chance to assess chemistry. You don't need to commit to a dinner on date 1, but go for the drink and maybe a shared appetizer or two. Alternatively, a lunch or weekend brunch is a little less formal, and you can incorporate a Moet or Bloody Mary into the mix if you desire. It just takes the edge off.

First Date Setting Matters: Choose Wisely

Third, don't choose a place where you frequent with your buddies. Carmela, a 59-year-old doctor, shared a frustrating first-date experience. Her date took her to a sports bar, ordered her a glass of wine, and then proceeded to focus on the game and chat with the bartender. It was an evening clearly centered around his interests, leaving Carmela feeling neglected and uncomfortable.

The Art of the First Date

For the first date, keep it simple. After the first date, you can get more creative with an activity and a little more levity—but the first date should be you and them in a standard setting. I had one client who lives in Southern California, in her mid-sixties. She matched with a guy, they planned a drink, and then all of sudden he changed his mind and wanted to take her to Disneyland.

I quickly chimed in no! Can you imagine being stuck with someone you just met for eight hours or so in long lines and in the hot sun? Better to avoid potential disaster.

**Consideration Counts:
Be Chivalrous**

Also, guys, let's pretend chivalry isn't dead for a second. Don't pick a place in your neighborhood that is really out of the way for your date. Take the initiative to figure out what works for her or find a place in between.

#60 Share Your Cell

**Simplify Communication
the Practical and Safe Way**

Unless you're Taylor Swift and somewhere in their known entity category, where messaging in the app is the way to go before getting to know a person, I recommend that 99.99 percent of the rest of us share our cell phone number before the first date.

This is for logistical purposes in case you and the other need to reach each other: running late or stuck in traffic— things I want you to do your best to avoid. Having each other's number is easier than having to go back on the dating app and being unsure if the message was received. And don't be afraid—if the other isn't your jam or on the odd/concerning side, BLOCK. It happens all the time and is not a big deal.

The Art of the First Date

#61 Prep: Stay Safe But Don't Ruin Potential Magic

**Resist the Urge:
Why Less Research Is Better**

Prior to a first date, less research is often better. You've read the profile, seen at least four photos, and know what they do for a living—so why not be spontaneous? Trust your gut and let the first impression happen in person. You're meeting in a safe, public place, and you've already told a friend or two when and where you're going. There's no need to Google everything—sometimes too much research can cloud your judgment.

Reflect on Your Reasons for Researching

If you feel compelled to dig deeper, ask yourself why. Is it just curiosity? A yellow flag? If it's a red flag, maybe reconsider the date altogether. Over-researching can lead to high expectations—something I always advise against. Let your date tell their story, not on the internet.

Andrea McGinty

A Note to Women: Breaking the Detective Habit

I'm addressing this mostly to women, as men rarely think about these things. Based on my experience working with over 30,000 people, women are more likely to feel the need to investigate. So, you're feeling uncertain about a guy before the date? Before diving into full detective mode, ask yourself why. Maybe you're 50/50 on him. Maybe he only has a couple of photos, and you're unsure if he's legit. Or maybe he's been online forever, and you wonder why. But remember, if you've seen him online all this time, what does that say about you, too?

When to Dive Deeper: Proceed With Caution

If you must dig deeper, here are a few options:

- **Google Lens**: Pop in his photo—95% of the time, this reveals his full name and online presence, such as LinkedIn or Facebook.

- **Freepeoplesearch.com**: An accurate (and free) way to find out more.

The Art of the First Date

- **Facebook Groups**: "Are We Dating the Same Guy?" is a popular group where people share info about men they've dated. However, keep in mind that some feedback could come from someone with a grudge, so use caution.

By this point, you might have spent more time researching than you will on the actual date—and you wonder why dating can feel so exhausting!

More Safety Tips

1. Keep personal info private: Before a first date, don't share your last name, home address, or workplace. (If your name is super unique and will easily come up in a search,

2. Create an anonymous username: If your name is unique, like Dagny or London, use something else for the app. This is common practice.

3. Super nervous? Consider a 10-minute video chat through the app. While I'm not a big fan of this (just go on the date!), it can help verify that they look like their photos and give a glimpse of their surroundings. The background can tell you a lot—like, is it a clean kitchen if they said they love cooking?

4. Meeting up: Always meet at the date venue—no one should pick anyone up.

5. Check-in with friends: Text one or two friends with details about your date: where, when, and the app you met them on.

6. Public spaces only: Stay in public—don't go hiking or anywhere secluded after a first drink.

7. Be mindful of what you share: Start slow and stay cautious. Avoid sharing too much personal information on the first date.

8. No home visits on dates 2 or 3: Keep it public.

9. Trust your gut: If you feel uncomfortable, leave. If you're uneasy, ask someone from the venue to walk you to your car or wait with you for an Uber.

10. Never send intimate photos: These could be used for blackmail or posted online. You don't know this person yet.

11. Don't share financial info: No need to give any sensitive information.

12. Stay sober: Stick to one drink to keep your judgment clear.

The Art of the First Date

13. Have an exit strategy: Always be prepared to leave if something feels off.

Staying safe while dating doesn't mean you need to overdo it on research. Trust your instincts and take things one step at a time.

#62 Dressing Appropriately

**The Downside of Coffee Dates:
Low Effort, Low Impact**

Another glaring reason I don't recommend coffee dates is that people don't make the effort to dress their best and put their best foot forward. Oftentimes, people will go straight from yoga in their sweaty clothes for a "quick coffee."

**Dress for Success:
Tailored and Thoughtful Outfits**

Dress appropriately for the weather and wherever it is you are going, but make sure it's one of the tailored, carefully curated outfits we discussed earlier. If you are going to summer dress, a nice dress for women or polo shirt for a man is recommended. (A collar, please!) An evening drink allows for a little more spunk if you want it. A nice suit if you're coming from work on a weekday, or a nice pair of heels to add some brevity to your outfit for the ladies works wonders.

Whatever you decide, make sure it's an outfit you've worn before and feel comfortable in.

Comfort is Key:
Wear What Works for You

The last thing you need is an itchy turtleneck or pants you need to keep pulling up, distracting you from the fun conversation.

#63 Be Punctual

Planning Ahead:
Ensuring You're On Time

Punctuality is paramount on a first date. Arriving on time demonstrates respect for your date's time and showcases your reliability. Arriving late can create a negative first impression and set a poor tone for the evening. It's pivotal to plan your route, account for potential traffic, and know the parking or Uber situation. A punctual person is often perceived as more confident and considerate.

The Art of the First Date

#64 The Sober Factor

**Keep Alcohol Discussions Light:
It's Not About the Drink**

Conversations about alcohol are boring and shouldn't be the centerpiece of the conversation, whether you drink or you don't drink. If you are sober for whatever reason (or your date is) no need to dwell.

**Avoiding Awkward Moments:
The Water Order Faux Pas**

But here is a big what *not* to do: I had one client who went for a first date drinks meet up and ordered water. Yikes. That is bound to make the other person feel awkward and gives the impression that they could just walk on out of there in 20 minutes, no tab and the dud at the party. Instead, ask for a cool mocktail, or an exotic juice.

If you drink and the date doesn't order one, so be it. Enjoy your beverage.

ANDREA MCGINTY

#65 Questions to Ask

Asking the right questions on a first date is the golden ticket to keep the conversation flowing and build rapport. Thoughtful inquiries not only demonstrate genuine interest but also provide opportunities for shared experiences and laughter, creating a foundation for a potential connection. Here are my recommendations to keep things light but moving (in no particular order!):

"Are You a Movie Fan?"
(Favorite Movie? Actor? Actress?)

It's always a fun topic, as most people are back to the movies or at least streaming. One date asked my client, *Top Gun* or *An Officer and a Gentleman?* Good question as *Top Gun 2* had just come out, and she went with *Top Gun*. He went with Officer as he thought the story about loyalty and growth was cool. She learned a little about him. Their favorite actress: they both chose Sandra Bullock and laughed. Definitely a second date here!

"So, What Do You Do for Fun?"

Easy, engaging question. You'll already know a bit about them from having read their profile: ski, SUP, tennis, opera, baseball games. So, it's easy to segue into a conversation. Note: You never have to have the exact same interests as you don't want a mirror image of yourself, right?

"What Do You Like to Read?"

Everyone reads something—whether it's the *Wall Street Journal, People Magazine, Huff Post,* or *National Geographic*. Easy topics are books. Funny how quite often I hear fiction fans are attracted to non-fiction fans, and vice versa. By concentrating on these types of hobby/action-oriented questions, you and your dates can promote a more positive, engaging, and enjoyable first-date experience. And, hopefully, a second date and more!

"Any Upcoming Vacations?"

Okay, who doesn't like to talk about travel? This question spirals into thoughts about favorite past vacations and bucket lists. You learn much from a person who climbed Denali to a person who likes the Cayman beach to an RV adventurer—their idea of adventure and activity.

Andrea McGinty

"Where'd You Grow Up?"

Many of us are not living where we grew up—this transitions into all the places a person has lived, their family and siblings, traditions, sports teams... just a fountain of information about your date! It's a simple, open-ended question that can lead to discussions about background, culture, and upbringing.

"You Had Great Photos–
Where Did You Take the One Scuba-diving?"

This question shows interest in the other's hobbies and experiences, leading to a potentially engaging story.

"What's the Best Concert You've Gone to?"
(Favorite films? Books?)

Why it's good: These questions delve into personal interests and can reveal shared passions, making the conversation livelier and more enjoyable.

The Art of the First Date

"Are You Having Fun with Online Dating?"

Yes, I encourage this question. Fun and online dating—stop laughing! Because it's a way of asking a much more important question—what we all really want to know, right? We want to know if they are a player, if they are serious about a relationship, if they just want to date, and if a whole slew of information comes your way.

Heather, a 52-year-old female in NYC (my client), asked her to date over drinks on Monday night. His reply? "You know, it's interesting—especially as an attorney, I tend to meet many bankers and other attorneys professionally. I'm looking for a long-term relationship with someone outside these professions. I mean, how else would I be sitting here with you—a fashion executive—I would have never met you. So, to answer your question, mostly it's been fun."

Wow did Heather learn a lot from this innocuous question! Yep, he was excited to be with her. Second date secured.   Asking this question can reveal a lot about someone's personality. Are they optimistic or pessimistic? Enthusiastic or burned out?

If someone asks you this question, I love the answer Janine uses: 'I'm having a blast meeting so many interesting men. I just haven't found the right one yet.' It's a great response because it shows confidence, desirability, and a positive outlook.

Keep the tone light and fun. Enjoy the date as you'll learn something new on each date. My client Josie went on a date with a personal trainer. She found quickly there wasn't much in common but she came away with some amazing new stretches to try! Also, discussing activities, music, or books can lead to discovering mutual interests, which is great for building a connection.

#66 Questions Not to Ask

Asking the wrong questions on a first date can quickly derail a promising connection. Inappropriate or overly personal inquiries can make someone feel uncomfortable, judged, or interrogated, creating awkwardness and hindering the development of rapport. Additionally, questions that reveal insensitivity or lack of understanding about current events or social issues can create a negative impression and hinder the possibility of a second date.

As a dating coach, where I talk to many clients weekly, sometimes I nearly fall off my office balance/exercise ball when they tell me what they discussed. Then they wonder, hmmm, why no second date?

So, here are the questions *not* to ask:

The Art of the First Date

"Tell Me about Yourself…"

It's vague and can make the date awkward, like the date must deliver a monologue or résumé. By the way, a client of mine got this question, and she began with: "I was born at 6:04 PM on Tuesday, May 9, 1971, at St. Luke Hospital in Philadelphia…. shall I go on?" Her date started laughing and said, sorry, that was a stupid question. The date just got better. Ice broken.

"What Was a Major Turning Point in Your Life that Got You Here?"

Excuse me! Aren't first dates light, fun, and casual? You've just basically asked: Tell me about your divorce, widowhood, bad breakups, and everything in between, which is intrusive and breaks every boundary of a first date. What are you —an executive recruiter?

"What's Your Relationship Like with Your Family?"

You're not addressing wedding invitations and trying to decide which weird sibling or uncle to exclude. Invasive, yep! You'll learn all this in time; be patient.

Andrea McGinty

"What's the Best Date You've Ever Had, and Why?"

Let's leave this with a short answer: I have no comment on this one, except perhaps that it was unbelievable.

"What Have You Learned about Yourself from Past Relationships?"

Yikes! You guaranteed no second date.

"When You're Feeling Down, What Always Cheers You Up?"

Well, you're not his/her therapist. Do you want to delve into something depressing on a first date?

"How Long Have You Been Using Dating Apps?"

This implies judgment and makes the date feel like a seasoned "dater," potentially creating discomfort or defensiveness. Who cares? Why would you care? Especially on a first date. It matters because...why? How does this affect whether you go on a second or third date or marry him/her?

The Art of the First Date

"How Do You Like Match, Bumble, Hinge, etc. So Far?"

This shifts the focus to the app rather than the person, often leading to negative rants. Nobody likes a Dating App until they meet someone.... then it's the greatest site in the world.

"What Are You Looking for?"

Ughhhh, way to put a person on the spot; plus, it makes you look desperate. It's too direct and makes the date feel like a job interview, putting unnecessary pressure on them. If you are unlucky and get this question, cut it off quickly with this: 'A second date with someone I like." Then, change the topic and move on to getting to know each other—books, film, music, activities, current events.

"Why Did Your Last Relationship End? Do You Have a Good Relationship with Your Ex?"

These questions are way too personal and can bring up negative emotions or stories, which is not conducive to a positive first-date atmosphere. A first date is nothing more than a precursor to a second date, hopefully, a third date, and so on. Yes, it will come up naturally, but this is not the time.

Andrea McGinty

"Are You Attracted to Me?"

I couldn't resist adding this one. Imagine being asked that bold question on a first date after just 20 minutes. I'm still reeling from the shock!

#67 More Things Your Date Doesn't Want to Hear

These will surprise you. Maybe not. But as a top dating coach, the stories I hear! What is a first date meant to be? Only a chance to see if you'd like a second date, not a therapy session. It's meant to be light, fun, and to see if you have a bit of chemistry and common topics.

Here are all-too-common topics in the 45-plus crowd I beg you steer clear of:

"Why the Split up (Divorce)– and in Particular–Who Initiated It?"

Think of it this way—you are at a dinner party or networking event, would you ever in a million years ask this question? Hopefully, no. Why do you care at this point? Now, this can become much more relevant after 4-5 dates; but at this point, there is interest on both sides, and you may have a brief chat about what occurred. Big first date no-no and a 100% guarantee you won't be seeing a second date with this person. Most of this will come out overtime, so please don't ask about it.

The Art of the First Date

Complaints (About Anything)

"A negative attitude drains, a positive attitude energizes."

Wow, this bodes well for happiness in the future, right? Wrong! Here are a few examples:

My client, Michael, 59, in NYC, met Lana for a lunch date on Tuesday. She walked in 10 minutes late, complained about her Uber driver, and how the rain had ruined her hair. The date went downhill from there. She proceeded to tell him about her arrogant boss and that she was thinking of changing jobs/careers. What were his thoughts? He told me, "She will be a nightmare to be in a relationship with," and he's one of the most positive guys I've had the pleasure of working with. Even Lana's good looks could not overcome her personality!

Ok, here's another one for the books.

Tim, 48, my client in Boca Raton met Annaliese for a drink. She immediately said she was famished, and did he mind if they ate dinner too? (Yes, he did as he just wanted to grab a drink and an appetizer and go to his son's soccer game after). Tim explained that he had another commitment afterwards and guess what she said? "Well, then, I hope you are at least paying for this date as it took me over an hour to get ready." Rude? I would say so. By the way, men don't care how long it took you to get ready. No one cares! Keep that to yourself.

Andrea McGinty

Physical Ailments

No, no, no! You have upcoming dental surgery or just got over a bad flu. Do you want to sound like a hypochondriac?

Political Rants

Ohhhhkkk. I won't touch this with a 10-foot pole. Isn't our country divisive enough as it is? Why would you want to start a fresh relationship and encounter with a person over this? Yes, you may feel strongly about this, and this is your right. It just does not show you in the most positive light. I didn't say a gentle conversation about the USA's state of affairs—I said a political rant! You just come across as angry, and it's not an appropriate conversation for a first meeting. Political discussions can come later. They have no place on a first date, and if a date does bring it up, I suggest: "Oh, I never talk politics, my ex or my kids on first dates. How about those Dodgers?" and laugh!

Problems with Children Or Family Conflicts

I think we'll just call this oversharing and inappropriate. This happened recently to Steve (my 64-year-old client meeting Tanya for the first time). She mentioned how upset she was that her 23-year-old daughter had cut her out of her life and then went on with why. Steve just told me afterwards, "Thank God it was a drink, and I was out of there in 30 minutes."

The Art of the First Date

He called me Friday afternoon to tell me about Karina—the antithesis of Tanya who was light and laughter, and they made plans to play disc golf tomorrow and he was excited.

Children's Schedules

There is no need to discuss children's schedules, doctors' appointments, special needs or anything of that nature on a first date. Sure, those things can enter the conversation down the line, but they are not appropriate first date material.

As a rule, avoid discussing anything you wouldn't be comfortable talking about to a random stranger at a cocktail party. I understand, we all have our difficulties in life, and I'm not saying you show up full of butterflies and rainbows. Isn't that why we have best friends to talk through our issues or a therapist? Think of your behavior on dates—don't you want to put your best foot forward? If you can't do this, hold off on dating until you can resolve some of your issues.

#68 How to Handle the "On the Apps" Question

The Classic Icebreaker That Needs to Go: Discussing the App

This one comes up all the time… and I can't wait for the day when it doesn't. You're having a nice drink at a cool bar by the water, and he or she says in what they think is breaking the ice: "So, how do you like Bumble or whatever the site you met on…"

What not to do is talk down (and this goes for the DMs too!).

"Oh, I hate it, I can't meet anyone decent. It feels like you are the first normal person I have met."

FAIL.

Keep it simple and upbeat.

"Oh, it's great. I've met lots of great and interesting people. I just haven't met the right one yet."

Change the topic, move on. Positive attitudes are gold.

#69 The Ex-Factor

**Leave Your Ex Out of It:
The First Date Rule**

Slipping your ex into the conversation is just, well, a turn-off on date number one. Don't mention him or her, don't refer, just keep it out of the equation for now. Your date doesn't need to know that your ex also likes Old Fashion's, or that she speaks 7 languages or that he is a brain surgeon or a billionaire. It's not relevant for now. Keep it out of the convo.

#70 Keeping on Your Best Behavior

It doesn't take a horror movie to scare off a potential partner. Sometimes, the smallest missteps can derail a promising first date. I've identified these common pitfalls that can easily be avoided.

Desperately Needy

Shocking, I know. Kevin, a 47-year-old CEO in Charlotte, told me last week about how an attractive woman revealed her desire to remarry within the first 15 minutes of their lunch date—primarily for medical benefits. Well, well, well, isn't that attractive?!

Looking Constantly at Your Phone

This is basic manners. If you're expecting an important call, inform your date immediately upon sitting down and explain why. Maybe your mom is in surgery, or a big deal is closing. We all have unavoidable interruptions. However, habitually checking your phone makes you appear anxious, self-important, or disrespectful of your date's time.

Talking Incessantly about Yourself

Yep, guys, I'm talking to you here. I hear this from over 50% of my female clients. Make sure you practice active listening and ask your date questions too.

The Art of the First Date

Tardy

Yes, traffic is a reality in LA, DC, Dallas, New York, San Francisco, Miami, and countless other cities—name any major city, and traffic is typically awful. Again, make sure you have your date's cell phone number and inform them if you'll be 5-10 minutes late. Most people are already nervous on first dates, so being late adds unnecessary stress. Arriving ten minutes early is considered on time. Plan accordingly because this could be the one.

Don't Drink More Than Two Cocktails

Never overindulge on a first date. Alcohol can lead to sloppiness and oversharing. And just repeating what I said earlier for good measure: if you're a non-drinker, order something other than water.

Andrea McGinty

#71 Body Language, Eye Contact, and Those Active Listening Skills

The Silent Communicator
Body language is crucial for creating a positive and engaging first impression. Maintaining eye contact, adopting an open posture, and actively listening demonstrate genuine interest and respect for your date. Conversely, crossing your arms, avoiding eye contact, or dominating the conversation can create a barrier and hinder connection. It's vital to balance sharing about yourself with actively listening to your date's stories. While it's important to be present and engaged, there's a fine line between active listening and oversharing. If a conversation takes an unexpected turn, it's perfectly acceptable to politely redirect the topic to maintain a comfortable and enjoyable atmosphere.

The Art of the First Date

#72 Building Up Your Conversation Skills

Conversation skills are requisite for building connection and understanding in dating, as they allow individuals to share thoughts, emotions, and experiences, fostering intimacy and compatibility. Effective communication also helps navigate potential conflicts and challenges, strengthening the foundation of a potential relationship. Let's refine this art a little more:

The "Spokes" Method

I'm a fan of this technique. Okay, think of a bicycle wheel. You have the hub, then the spokes. Imagine you're on a first date; he mentions he's a huge football fan and starts talking about the Patriots and the great loss of Tom Brady a few years ago. You know absolutely nothing about football, Tom Brady, and you're not from Boston. He's in the hub—you jump to the spoke. "Oh, I grew up in Toronto where hockey was the sport. Ever been to a hockey game?" You easily steered the conversation away from just football without acknowledging your football ignorance. This strategy works for many topics!

Andrea McGinty

Interrupt Politely

Last week, my client Amelia was on a first date with a pilot who went on and on for 20 minutes about flying. She jumped in during a tiny pause in the conversation and said, "Wow, I feel like I know so much about you. What would you like to know about me?" It worked—and saved the date!

Listen Actively

Nope, you're not thinking about what you are going to say next because you are present.

Read into Sentences

Kayla comments over a beer on a first date, "Oh, I pray it doesn't rain tomorrow as I have a pickleball match then a pool party." She just told you a few things about herself: a) she plays pickleball, b) using the word "pray" suggests she might have a belief in God or religion, and c) she is social.

The Art of the First Date

Use Tone

Yes, words tell us quite a bit, but the tone conveys excitement, boredom, frustration, happiness, and much more.

Don't Hesitate

A pause is fine, but you want to exude confidence. Confidence is sexy!

Scan the News

Current events are always a good topic for first dates. Especially positive or unique stories. Remember my favorite **https://join1440.com...** It is simple and free!

Use Facial Expressions

Crucial—except in a game of poker! A smile goes a long way.

Engage

He's a computer nerd (and you're not)—an easy question is "What do you think of AI?"

Emphasize

Sometimes people mix this term up with sympathy. Empathy is simply the ability to understand and share the feelings of another.

Be Concise

Okay, we all tell stories, but a long rambling story is a bore.

Use the "Fact Disclosure"

Share a little bit of information about yourself, but nothing you wouldn't like to see quoted about you the next day online/Facebook/Instagram.

Sincere Compliments

These reap benefits and can set the other person at ease. "Oh, I love your sunglasses—may I ask where you got them?" Stay away from looks—I can't tell you how many online compliments I see that are "Wow, you're gorgeous" or "Great body—you must work out a lot"— Yuk. And ick.

What to Do Prior to a Date on an Online Dating Site…

I have a female client, Sonya, who is quite accomplished in the business realm. While her profile talked a bit about her career, it was by no means boastful. Sonya had several messages from men complimenting her on her business success. The guy who got her? A marketing executive named Drew. Here was his message: **"**Wow, I loved hearing about your yearly family reunions; how do you get 7 siblings to agree on the venue? That's quite an accomplishment"!
 Sonya loved that comment— she and Drew have been together a year now.

The Art of the First Date

Use Body Language

The stats are something like—80% of communication is body language, 20% words. Fidgeting with your phone, looking around the room, poor eye contact, and crossed arms are all signs that you are uncomfortable and don't want to be there.

#73 Who Pays?

Navigating the Etiquette

I'll keep this simple. It's what is comfortable and there are regional differences. For example, I see much splitting of the cost in NYC and LA. In the south? Not a chance; the men insist on paying for the most part. Call me old-fashioned, but men should pay for the first date. This doesn't mean the woman should just sit there when the check arrives (at least reach for your purse and offer genuinely to contribute). But guys, if you want a second date, pay the tab and do so quietly without fanfare and making a deal of it. Ladies, say thank you. Don't take this for granted. On same sex dates, who first asked should pay. Otherwise, if it was a joint decision to meet, split the tab.

Andrea McGinty

#74 How to End the Date Gracefully

Deciphering the End-of-Date Talk: What It Really Means

This can sometimes be an awkward sticky point. Perhaps you can't wait to go on a second date, but you aren't sure if the other feels the same? Or, one date was enough, or maybe you are on the fence whether you'd like to see this person again. For you 50-50 daters, my advice is always: Go. What do you have to lose but an hour or two of your time?

Remember: the majority of people in their 30s through 60s didn't experience instant fireworks on their first date; yet many ended up in happy relationships. Regardless, ending a first date on a positive note is important, whether you're interested in a second date or not. Don't send mixed signals. Your words can significantly influence the outcome and ensure both parties leave with a clear understanding of each other's intentions.

The Art of the First Date

10 Common End-the-Night Phrases

Here are ten common phrases people use at the end of a first date, along with some insights:

1. "I had a great time tonight." This clear and positive statement indicates interest in seeing the person again.

2. "I'd love to do this again sometime." While well-intentioned, "sometime" can be ambiguous. For clarity, consider specifying a desired activity or time frame.

3. "Thank you for a wonderful evening." This phrase, while polite, can sound overly formal and lacks specificity.

4. "I really enjoyed getting to know you." A versatile option that expresses appreciation for the company without making specific commitments.

5. "I hope you have a great rest of your week." A polite but distant ending, suggesting limited interest in future interactions.

6. "Let's stay in touch." A good option if you're open to future possibilities but not ready to commit to a second date.

7. "I appreciate your company tonight." This phrase can sound impersonal and lacks enthusiasm.

8. "It was nice meeting you." A classic choice for ending a date without interest in pursuing a relationship.

8. "I'm not sure we're a match, but I enjoyed our time together." Honest and kind, this statement provides clarity without causing hurt.

9. "Would you be interested in doing this again?" This direct approach shows confidence and clearly expresses interest in a second date.

Honesty and clarity are key to successful first date endings. Choose your words carefully to convey your true feelings and intentions. It's a simple, open-ended question that can lead to discussions about background, culture, and upbringing.

#75 Why You Might Not Want to Bother With Date 2

Oftentimes, the chemistry just isn't there on a first date. Perhaps you didn't have a great time or struggled to keep the conversation flowing. The reality is, it's unlikely to improve. Most singles are on their best behavior during an initial meeting, so if you're picking up negative vibes from the start, it's time to move on. With 128 million singles in the US, there's no need to settle!

Common Signals to "Cease and Desist"

Here are some common flashing signals that might indicate you shouldn't pursue a second date:

1. Excessive baggage: Doug, a 45-year-old CFO, recently described a date with a woman who seemed great online. She arrived 15 minutes late, apologized, then immediately launched into a rant about her babysitter's problems, followed by complaints about her ex-partner's lack of child support. It's unlikely that her life will become less stressful in the near future.

2. Anger management issues: A huge warning sign. Lana, 53, was on a dinner date when her companion became enraged over an incorrect drink order. He spoke rudely to the waiter and demanded to see a manager. This type of behavior is unacceptable and should be a deal-breaker.

3. Questionable questioning techniques: Either asking too many questions or asking none at all can be off-putting. Rapid-fire questioning can feel invasive, while a complete lack of curiosity suggests disinterest or narcissism. Balanced conversation involving both parties is key for a successful first date.

4. Incompatible sense of humor: If you don't find your date's jokes funny, it's unlikely their humor will change.

5. Excessive drinking: While enjoying a drink or two is common on first dates, excessive alcohol consumption can be an ominous indicator. It can lead to inappropriate behavior or create a negative impression.

6. Distracted behavior: Constant phone checking, looking around the room, or lack of eye contact indicates disinterest and disrespect. It's fundamental for both parties to be fully present during a date.

7. Unpunctuality without apology: Arriving late without a prior explanation shows a lack of respect for your time. While occasional delays can be understandable, chronic lateness is a red flag.

While second chances can sometimes work, it's important to trust your instincts and prioritize basic manners and respect. If a first date doesn't feel right, there's no need to force a connection. Focus on finding someone who shares your values and interests.

#76 Get Familiar with What Men Don't Want in Early Dating

In a recent poll of my male clients, these issues emerged as the most significant indicators of trouble and complaints. But hang on, guys, you're not off the hook— I detail women's complaints about men in online dating next!

This poll focused on all aspects of online dating, from initial online encounters to up to five in-person dates. The 742 male participants ranged in age from 35 to 65 and were all active online daters.

Misrepresenting Physical Attributes.

Men reported that women often misrepresented their age, physical appearance, or both. Interestingly, 68% of men said they would still have agreed to a first date even if they had known the woman's accurate details upfront. However, 59% declined a second date primarily due to these discrepancies.

Premature Deep Dives into the Past

An overwhelming number of men reported being asked about their divorce or past relationships on the first date. While brief inquiries about relationship status or children were acceptable to most, detailed questions about the reasons for divorce were considered inappropriate and off-putting. Many men felt these discussions were better suited for later stages of a relationship.

Financial Expectations

While not explicitly a complaint, 81% of men reported paying for the first date. They suggested that women express gratitude and their interest in a second date within 24 hours, regardless of their ultimate decision.

Lack of Initiative

Over 75% of men expressed frustration with women who simply send likes, winks, or smiles without initiating a conversation. They felt that women should put in equal effort by sending a brief message to start a dialogue.

Vague Dating Suggestions

Men appreciated when women took initiative in suggesting specific date ideas, such as a particular restaurant or activity. They found the phrase "want to grab coffee or lunch sometime" to be vague and lacking in enthusiasm. Conversely, suggesting a specific time and place demonstrated interest and confidence.

#77 Get Familiar with What Women Don't Want in Early Dating

A poll of 836 women aged 38-67 revealed these common grievances in online dating:

Misrepresented Height

While the average American man is 5'9", many online profiles exaggerate height by two to three inches. It's common to find:

The Art of the First Date

1. A man claiming 5'8" is likely 5'6".
2. A man claiming 5'9" is likely 5'7" or 5'8".
3. A man claiming 5'10" is likely 5'8" or 5'9".
4. A man claiming 6'1" is probably over 6'.
5. Men claiming 6'2" or taller are generally accurate.

Stale Dating Profiles

Many men maintain outdated online profiles. Perhaps they created their profile years ago and haven't updated their photos, age, or career information.

Lack of Response to Messages

While some men might be inactive on dating apps, women often find it challenging to initiate and maintain engaging conversations. Crafting thoughtful and personalized messages can significantly increase response rates.

Love Bombing

This overwhelming display of attention and affection early in a relationship can be alarming. It's vital to maintain boundaries and proceed cautiously when encountering such behavior.

Ghosting

Disappearing without explanation is disrespectful and hurtful. A brief, polite message ending the connection is always preferable to ghosting.

These findings highlight shared challenges women face in the online dating purview. By addressing these issues, both men and women can improve their dating experiences.

#78 Following Up Afterwards

Modern Etiquette:
Embracing Prompt Follow-Ups

Gone are the days of rigid post-date etiquette. The old rulebook of waiting three days to follow up is outdated. In today's connected world, it's perfectly acceptable to express your interest or disinterest promptly. If you had a wonderful time, a thank-you text that same evening, expressing gratitude for the date and excitement for a potential next outing, is appropriate and confident.

Politely Declining:
Clear and Courteous

Conversely, if you're not interested, a polite and brief message the following day acknowledging the date, but declining further interest is respectful and necessary. Timely communication demonstrates good manners and clarity, benefiting both parties involved. Ladies, you don't need to wait for the man to text first! Showing initiative and confidence, especially if you are keen for date 2, is pretty darn sexy.

#79 Assessing the Connection

**The 1-100 Scale:
An Analytical Approach to
Assessing Romantic Potential**

I'm a woman of numbers. To assess the potential of a romantic connection, I employ a simple yet effective one-to-hundred scale. A score of one indicates absolutely no interest, while a hundred represents a perfect match. Realistically, most people will fall somewhere in the middle. This numerical approach helps to remove emotional biases and provides a clearer perspective.

**Applying the Scale:
Making Strategic Dating Decisions**

By assigning a number to a potential partner, whether after seeing their profile or following a first date, it becomes easier to determine next steps. A score above 50 warrants a second date to explore the connection further. Conversely, a score below 50 suggests that pursuing the relationship may not be worthwhile. This system encourages a more strategic approach to dating, allowing individuals to make informed decisions based on objective criteria rather than impulsive feelings.

Andrea McGinty

#80 If You Had a Plain Weird Date, Just Know You Aren't Alone

**Unforgettable First Dates:
Tales from the Wild Side**

Sometimes, strange dates happen. The kind of dates so out there that you really cannot make them up. And I've had a front-row seat to the dating world's wildest moments for the past 30 years. Here's what some clients have shared about their unforgettable first dates:

1. Jon, 47, Boulder, CO: We embarked on a "walk and talk" date—a refreshing change from the usual coffee shop monotony. Our coffee run took a surprising turn when she led me to a cemetery filled with headstones dating back to the 1800s. She then proceeded to sob uncontrollably at random gravesites. Despite her beauty, this morbid behavior was a deal-breaker.

2. Thomas, 55, Las Vegas: Our second date was at the opulent Caesar's Palace buffet. I was astonished by her appetite as she returned for thirds, piling her plate high with food. Normally, I'd applaud such enthusiasm, but this was on another level. To top it off, she casually mentioned she'd just stopped taking Ozempic after losing 75 pounds and was eager to tackle the dessert spread.

3. Amy, 49, Los Angeles: We were from distinct parts of the country and happened to be in Salt Lake City, Utah at the same time. He asked to meet in between work "meetings" at a nearby hospital. It turned out he was traveling to collect donor organs, which is what he does all over the country. I learned about a whole industry that I knew in the back of my mind existed, but really never put two and two together that it's a profession, too.

4. Atticus, 52, Dallas: Our first date was at a sophisticated wine bar in Preston Center. Given her professed love for rodeo and horses, I braced myself for a hint of country charm. Instead, I was hit with a wave of barn odor as she walked in. The heat, combined with the smell, caused a neighboring couple to discreetly move down the bar.

5. Kevin, 66, NYC: We met for drinks near Times Square, and she warned me she'd be in her work attire. Little did I know she meant "lion costume." Yes, a fully costumed lion sat down beside me, claiming to be a fan. The evening was certainly memorable, and I even got offered a ticket to the Lion King.

6. Michael, 67, Laguna Beach: Our first date was a windsurfing adventure. Given her impressive online resume of water sports, I was excited. Reality quickly set in as she struggled to control the sail and was swept away from me. Thankfully, the Coast Guard came to the rescue. After that, I opted for more traditional first dates.

7. Megyn, 60, Charleston: He wanted to meet at the mall for our first date. I figured we would grab a bite, perhaps walk around. No, the date told me I was the same height and size as his sister and asked if I could try some clothes on so he could buy her a Christmas present. I tried one dress on, and then felt ridiculous as this guy I didn't know assessed me. I left. I also suspected the gift wasn't for his sister.

If something strange happens that makes you want to throw in the towel, take a deep breath, laugh it off, and know that you certainly aren't alone. Onward and upward.

The combination of yellow and green is **CHARTREUSE,** a gentle progression, representing growth and potential. **From First Date to Second… and Beyond.**

chapter 7
From First Date to Second... and Beyond

#81 Planning Date 2

**Leveling Up:
Date 2 Should Be Memorable**

You both agree to date 2? Awesome. Let's shake things up! Repeating the same old drinks routine is a snooze fest. Think creatively. Plan an activity that's short, fun, engaging, and gives you both a chance to connect.

A short morning bike ride followed by coffee (coffee doesn't bother me in this date 2 context because you have time together), a fun museum visit with a post-tour bite, or even a casual stroll through a park at sunset or even a movie followed by dinner can be a refreshing change of pace. The goal is to create new experiences and keep the spark alive.

From First Date to Second... and Beyond

Fun, Not Overly Committed

However, I stress that the activity should be relatively short—no all-day Disneyland passes or fifteen-mile hikes. You know what I mean. Also, an activity can be a terrific way to test your date on the BS scale. One of my client's, who loves biking, would always opt for a nice beach trail Sunday ride—and could immediately tell whether that oft-reciprocated "I love biking too!" was a true statement. So, that was a good measuring stick for him.

Other fun ideas include a comedy club, ax throwing, bowling, or hanging out at a fabulous vintage bookstore. (A few of my New York clients love The Strand bookstore if both are into reading!) If you both love music, why not find a cool local band that is playing?

#82 Mind Your Manners

The Little Things Make a Big Impression

If date number 1 was just drinks, there is a good chance date number 2 will involve food… Keep in mind, good manners never go out of style. Even if you've been flying solo for a while, it's important to remember that little things like not inhaling your food like a starving wolf or knowing which fork to use can make an enormous difference. And guys, pulling out that chair and holding the door? Total classic. It's not just about being polite; it shows you care and that you respect the other person. Trust me, it goes a long way.

Andrea McGinty

#83 Keep Multiple Dates In Rotation

**Avoiding the One-Basket Syndrome:
Keep Your Options Open**

Keeping your options open is key in the preliminary stages of dating. It's easy to get caught up in someone and put all your eggs in one basket when you really like someone, but it's important to stay on the apps and to go forth in meeting new people. I can't tell you the number of times clients have told me they've met a special someone and don't want to date others, only to learn later that the other person has continued to date other people and eventually falls for someone else!

**A Balanced Approach:
Enjoy the Journey Without Pressure**

The moral of the tale: continue to explore your options until you and your potential partner have a clear understanding of exclusivity. By juggling a few dates at once, you increase your chances of finding a great match and protect yourself from disappointment. Dating should be fun, so enjoy the process and don't put unnecessary pressure on yourself. It all comes down to numbers, so be strategic about it. Maybe you have three dates scheduled this week—one is a first date, another is date 2, and the third one flaked and fell out of the picture. But keep the flow going. You aren't exclusive until you both make that clear commitment.

From First Date to Second... and Beyond

#84 The Block Hack

**Clean Up Your Feed:
The Power of Blocking**

If you keep seeing the same unwanted profiles on your dating app, don't hesitate to block them. This simple action can significantly improve your online dating experience by preventing repeated encounters with people you're not interested in. Maintaining a clean profile and being organized can also streamline your search. When it comes to online dating, your options are straightforward: either connect or block.

#85 The 3-Date Barometer

**The Three-Date Rule:
Giving Connections a Fair Chance**

Okay, you've met someone interesting, and the sparks might be flying. Great! Or more commonly, you just aren't quite sure how you feel. More often than not, it takes a few interactions to get a true sense of someone

But before you cross them off the list completely because you wanted fireworks and shooting stars in your stomach, consider the three-date rule. Give it three dates to assess compatibility and chemistry. That gives you enough of a chance to assess whether the two of you have potential. If, after that time, you're still unsure about the connection, it's probably a no.

When Distance is a Factor

Distance can play a role. If you live far apart, it might take longer to build a strong connection. The key is to enjoy the process, keep an open mind, and trust your instincts.

#86 Date 3 Complete? Red Flags To Be Aware Of

Sometimes, you won't see a red flag on the first date. Both singles are on their best behavior, and the date is great. But by date 3, you should be to tell if there are some issues that will be future deal-breakers. After over 30 years as a dating coach and providing online dating services, you'd be surprised by what pops up on dates 2 and 3.

From First Date to Second... and Beyond

Red Flags That Surface by Date 3: Knowing What to Watch For

Here are 10 to pay attention to:

1. Right Person, Wrong Time Darn it, it happens! You may have met the right man—but he just finished a long divorce or is recovering from being widowed. She may be the right woman—but she's stressed with a new job, caring for an ailing parent, or just had a major life event such as moving or a death. Six months later, this person might be "the one," but they are not the "right one now."

2. No Follow Through: Haven't we all had that first date where we just clicked and made plans for a second date? Then… nothing. You don't hear from her for weeks; when you do, it's a lame excuse. Or you made plans for a game of tennis, and an hour before, he cancels with no reason. Consistency builds trust, and trust builds a relationship.

3. No Questions: You're both attracted to each other—and all he does is talk, talk, talk. About himself. His work. His golf game. He asks you no questions. Let's say this occurred on date 1. Date 2 begins in the same fashion. What would I advise? Graciously cut into the conversation with, "Wow, Michael, I feel like I know so much about you. Ok, so what would you like to know about me? Fire away." If he doesn't get the hint, adios.

4. Venting: Oh, what fun is this. A major sign of negativity—who needs this? Whether she's venting about online dating (run), her son's college tuition and how the ex pays nothing, the ex, the weather—well, she is showing her true colors. Maybe she's having a difficult day. Nope, that's just an excuse. Don't we all want positivity in our lives? If this is the beginning of a potential relationship, just imagine how much worse it will get. I don't care how good-looking she (or he) is!

5. Distracted: No eye contact. Playing with her cell phone. Looking around the room. Looking at his watch. Asking you to repeat a question. I could go on and on with this one.

6. Avoiding: You are on a date, and they are evasive about basic questions like what they do professionally, family, where they live. Now, I don't mean you should be asking super personal questions like "When was your last relationship?" or "Are you looking for a long-term relationship?" as those are inappropriate for the first 1 or 2 dates. I'm thinking right now of some of my clients that are in long-term relationships—the first few dates were about common interests, current events, travel, etc.

From First Date to Second... and Beyond

7. Constant Texting: Lara, a 45-year-old client of mine, really liked Chris after the first 2 dates. But then he began texting constantly—every few hours. As an ER doc, it annoyed her. She told him, "Please, no texting during the day." You know his response? "I miss you." Needy, I daresay, and she correctly moved on—and is now happily dating a "normal" texter!

8. Hot and Cold: One moment they are warm, the next they've seemingly forgotten about you.

9. Can't Plan Anything: Two facets to this one: great first date, then endless texting, and he/she can't plan anything because of a bunch of insipid excuses—work's really busy, I have a seminar this weekend, my friend is in town, I'll get back to you. This is not what you want—so don't put up with this, move on.

It's the 2020s. To be fair, it's up to both people to produce fun dating ideas. He might suggest bike riding—like my client Hunter did on his date on Saturday—they rode over 14 bridges in NYC and had a blast. His date suggested a trivia night this week. The worst? "What would you like to do?" answered with, "Oh, I'm easy—you pick."

10. Talks About Money Rich man, poor man. Either way, boasting about how much you make, your toys, your 5-star vacations—just makes you look insecure. On the other hand, "I'm underpaid," "My wife took all in the divorce," "My ex refuses to pay child support"—all are inappropriate and particularly good signals to move on.

Andrea McGinty

#87 How To Handle The First Month Of Dating

Pacing Yourself:
Slow Is Smooth, and Smooth is Fast

1. Go slow. Perhaps by week 3, you're up to 2 dates per week, and by week 8, 3 dates per week, including overnight stays.

2. There's no formula or expectation for a sleepover. It could be date 3 or month 3.

3. Limit texts to one per day or every other day during the first two weeks. Avoid appearing too eager. Too much, too soon can be a major turn-off.

4. Avoid introducing family members too soon.

5. Consider a party with friends around week 3 after a few dates. This will allow you to observe their interactions with your friends and assess their confidence level.

6. Don't focus solely on eating or drinking during the first month. Try other activities like biking, pickleball, hiking, walking, boating, or attending a movie. One of my favorite first-month dates was visiting a bookstore after a film and discussing our purchases over wine. This can be a fun way to learn more about each other.

From First Date to Second... and Beyond

7. Never cancel plans at the last minute unless it's a true emergency. Rain and your hair are not valid excuses.

8. Avoid making long-term plans.

9. Don't come on too strong or reveal your must-haves in a relationship too early.
Don't neglect your friends and personal interests.

10. Be authentic. Be yourself, not a version you think they might prefer. How long could you maintain a facade?

#88 Looking For This to Last Long-Term? More on What Not to Do

My clients range in age from 28 to 78 years old—and all ages in between. If any of these behaviors show up in your first 3 encounters, let's face it—they will only get worse. You may know my saying: "The best behavior is in the first month(s) of dating.

Andrea McGinty

**The "Ex Factor":
When Past Relationships Linger Too Long**

Daniel, a successful 58-year-old attorney and client of mine, recapped this story for me. It was his second date with Anna, a pretty 57-year-old teacher in Oregon. They'd just had a pleasant tapas and sangria-fueled dinner, and he was driving her home. She took a phone call from her ex-husband in the car, something to do with one of their children. (That's okay, right?). The small incident was resolved in five minutes, but then she launched into a story with her ex: "Remember when we…" and for the next 20 minutes of the car ride home, she reminisced with her ex in front of Daniel.
Think there was a third date? She texted him, surprised he never asked her out again.

1. Talking on the Phone While on a Date If it's not an emergency or important, why? You just showed your date you don't value their time.

2. Too Inquisitive Nosy. Of course, we are talking about the first 3 dates here. Sure, you can ask how long someone has been divorced. But the buck stops there. It's none of your business at this point why they divorced, if it was acrimonious, or if they're paying a hefty alimony, etc. Mark, 45, told me a woman asked him if he ever cheated on his wife—on the first date. He was new to online dating and asked me if that was normal. Heck, no!

From First Date to Second... and Beyond

3. Bad Relationships with Family and They Tell You About It Maria, 37, had a date last week with Mark over coffee. Within 10 minutes, he told her he was estranged from his children because he was never present in their lives. As he began launching into his dysfunctional childhood, she drained her latte and told him this wasn't going to work in a gracious manner. He looked confused. He texted her the next day asking what he did wrong, and while tempted to tell him he needed a whole lot of therapy, she just said she felt no connection. Smart. There is absolutely no reason to stay for an hour when someone launches their issues on you. (Oh, she blocked him on her phone too). Things like this—you just move on!

4. Language Okay, so she's a Wall Street trader and exposed to foul language—and uses it herself. As Michael commented, "I walk in, see this pretty, petite woman and think, yes! Then she opened her mouth."

5. They Don't Make You Laugh Many people comment in online profiles that they enjoy a sense of humor. But that can range from silly, goofy, quirky to a jokester. You either click on this—or don't! And I have to add—do you make them laugh? I had a client in Chicago, who told me none of her dates were funny. I asked her if she was funny, and she said "no." Discussion over.

6. Gossipy On first few dates? You don't even know this person very well yet. Now, I'm not talking about telling funny stories; I'm talking about a mean-spirited way of describing people. Talking badly about others does not resonate with the majority of people.

7. Talking Negatively About Your Dating App/ Dates You've Gone On I will keep drumming this down because it matters… optimism. Laura, a positive and happy-go-lucky client of mine, shared this story with me. Her date's first question was, "Are you finding these dating sites as awful as I am?" She was surprised and I liked her answer: "Wow, really. I've met some fantastic men—just not the right one for me yet." And guess what? Even after her comment, he wanted to continue talking about all the unattractive women he'd met. She immediately tossed him out of her line-up of potential second dates.

8. Bad Manners Christopher, 64, had invited Louisa on a date to a wine bar for one drink. When he arrived, she was on her second glass of wine and busy ordering not one, but three appetizers. He gave her the benefit of the doubt, but when the check appeared, she left to make a phone call. Now, Christopher is a gentleman who always pays the check, but he was perplexed when she didn't even bother saying thank you. She had scarfed down most of the appetizers and ordered a third drink too.

From First Date to Second... and Beyond

9. Drinks Too Much Well, I guess #8 covered this one!

10. And the Good Old Rude to the Waitstaff Definitely shows one's true colors. Laura met Thomas for a third date at Mastro's, a nice steakhouse in Newport Beach. (Prior to that, they'd had a pleasant coffee meeting). First, he complained about his salad. But the denouement came when he angrily chastised the waiter about the temperature of his steak and asked to speak to a manager.

Keep in mind most of the time I hear fun, heart-warming stories about the first few dates. Sure, not everyone has chemistry, and it's not always love at first sight. But if you spot the above "red flags" on the first three encounters, chances are it will not get better.

My clients who do best and add to my 65% success rate of developing relationships tend to be positive, well-mannered singles. It only takes one, so don't give up after one unpleasant experience. With 128 million singles alone in the US, I promise he/she may be right around the corner. Chalk it up to experience—and move on to that next date!

#89 Keep The Momentum Alive

The Honeymoon Phase: Beyond the Initial Spark

The first month/honeymoon phase of dating is all fun and games, right? Everyone's on their best behavior, and it feels like magic. Yet, let's be real, that initial spark needs to evolve into something more substantial. To give yourselves the best chance of success, plan activities and dates you both enjoy (don't fall into the humdrum of dinner/drinks every time!) But with that, plenty of quality talking time is pivotal, too.

Building Real Connections: Consistency and Proximity Matter

Seeing someone regularly is key to building a real connection. It's like testing out a new car: you need to take it for a spin to see if it handles well in different conditions. Long-distance relationships can be super exciting at first, but the lack of face-to-face time can create an unrealistic image of the other person. It's like watching a highlight reel without seeing the bloopers. So, if possible, aim for something closer to home—that is, stay away from long-distance lure—to get a true sense of compatibility.

From First Date to Second... and Beyond

#90 The Vacation Test: A Real-life Reality Check

**Relationship Milestone:
The Power of a Shared Getaway**

Taking a vacation together (or just an extended weekend away) can be a major relationship milestone. It's a condensed version of everyday life, packed with potential stressors and quality time. You'll quickly see how you handle conflicts, compromise, and spending extended periods together. Think of it as a crash course in compatibility. Of course, not every trip is a disaster, but it can certainly reveal hidden aspects of someone's personality.

**The Real Test:
Navigating Unexpected Challenges**

Even though it's exciting to plan that dream getaway, it's important to approach it with realistic expectations and a keen eye. Vacations can make or break, and a great test whether this really will work. It's also a valuable ascertain when things don't go to plan. Flight delayed for 7 hours? Hotel overbooked? Observing how your partner responds to life's curveballs can get you a sense (for better or for worse) whether this is the person for you.

However, don't hurry into this too early in the dating process. You want to feel as secure as possible in the presence of the other—you're likely sharing a bathroom, don't forget—before entering into long stretches together.

#91 Signs It's All-Moving Right

Ah, one of life's great challenges—how to read the signals that he or she is falling for you. Pretty basic, you think, right? But you wouldn't believe the number of women (men too) I talk to weekly as part of my online dating coaching that say "Hey, Andrea, what do you think? Does he like me?" Quite often this is after the 3rd, 5th, 10th date with the same person!

While there's no foolproof guide, certain behaviors often signal deeper interest. Let's start with some of the male signs:

1. Prioritizing You.
A man who consistently is available for you and prioritizes your happiness is likely invested in the relationship. Look for actions that demonstrate he values your time and company.

2. Future Planning
Incorporating you into future plans, whether it's a casual mention of a potential event or a more concrete invitation, suggests he sees you as a long-term possibility.

From First Date to Second... and Beyond

3. Introducing You to His Circle
Meeting his friends or family is a significant step. It shows he's comfortable with the idea of you being a part of his life.

4. Vulnerability and Openness
Sharing personal thoughts, feelings, and experiences demonstrates trust and emotional intimacy.

5. Physical Affection
While not exclusive to romantic relationships, increased physical touch, such as holding hands or cuddling, can signal deeper connection.

6. Consistent Communication
Regular and meaningful communication, whether through texts, calls, or in-person interactions, indicates interest and investment.

While men often express interest more directly, women tend to be more subtle. Here are three common non-verbal signs to watch for:

1. Eye Contact: Prolonged eye contact often indicates interest.

2. Body Language: Open posture, leaning in, and mirroring your actions can be positive signs.

3. Touch: Accidental or intentional touches can signal attraction.

Here are some four common verbal signs to watch for:

1. Active Listening: She pays attention to what you say and asks thoughtful questions.
2. Laughter: Genuine laughter at your jokes is a good indicator of enjoyment.

3. Sharing Personal Information: Revealing personal details often signifies trust and interest.

4. Compliments: She finds ways to compliment you, both physically and personally.

Here are three behavioral clues to be on the lookout for:

1. Initiating Contact: If she's the one reaching out first, it's a strong sign of interest.

2. Making Plans: Suggesting activities or future plans shows she's interested in spending more time with you.

3. Remember Details: If she remembers intricate details about your life, it suggests she's paying attention.

These are broad-stroke indicators, and individual behavior can vary. Trust your instincts and enjoy the process of getting to know someone new.

From First Date to Second... and Beyond

#92 Signs It Is Time to Move On

Navigating the complexities of modern dating can be challenging, but recognizing warning signs early on can save you time and heartache. Here are some common warning signs to watch out for:

1. One-Sided Effort. If you're consistently initiating plans, putting in more effort, or feeling like you're carrying the relationship, it might be time to reassess. A healthy partnership involves mutual investment.

2. Lack of Communication. Effective communication is the foundation of any successful relationship. If your partner avoids difficult conversations or struggles to express their feelings, it could be a sign of deeper issues.

3. Lack of Chemistry. Sometimes, it just doesn't click. There's no way to force a connection. Richard, for example, enjoyed talking to Aria and found her interesting, but he wasn't attracted to her physically. In such cases, it's best to move on.

4. Inconsistent Behavior. Hot and cold behavior can be incredibly confusing and emotionally draining. If someone is constantly canceling plans or disappearing without explanation, it's likely they're not fully invested.

5. Disrespectful or Inconsiderate Actions. This includes anything from belittling your feelings to disregarding your boundaries. Healthy relationships are built on mutual respect.

6. Negative Outlook. Someone who consistently focuses on the negative or has a pessimistic worldview can bring down your mood. A positive and optimistic outlook is essential for a fulfilling partnership.

These are just some common cautionary signals, and every relationship is unique. Trust your instincts and prioritize your happiness.

#93 Dodge The Dating Dilemmas

I've witnessed a range of challenges that women face in the dating world. For example, when Carol, a 47-year-old architect from Dallas, came to me last month, she was frustrated that she hadn't yet met "the one" after being online for a year.
Here's what I found:

1. **Issue #1.** She believed each man she met over the last six months was "the one" after just the first date.

2. **Issue #2.** Carol expressed that she was falling in love after each initial encounter.

While Carol is a positive and intelligent woman, her tendency to fall in love too quickly was more reflective of unrealistic expectations than genuine connection. Falling in love after the first date? That's more like a Hallmark movie than real life!

Common Dating Mistakes to Avoid
So, let's jump into some common dating mistakes people make:

1. **Looking for a Perfect Partner.** In my coaching sessions, I often see clients nitpick potential matches. He's an inch too short, he rides horses, or his hair is receding—these critiques can be overly harsh. Remember, it's rare to find someone online who fits your ideal perfectly. Instead, focus on the ones that intrigue you—those "50/50" profiles that could lead to great first dates.

2. **Talking About Medical Issues.** Unless you show up with an arm cast from a pickleball incident, there's no need to discuss your health history. First dates should be fun, not a medical consultation.

3. Pretending to Be Interested in Things You're Not. Lauren, 39, went on a date with Jerry, who was excited about his recent golf trip to Scotland. To keep the conversation flowing, she pretended to love golf, even mentioning she was thinking of taking lessons. When he texted for a second date, she panicked and asked, "How do I get out of this golf thing?" Authenticity is key—be yourself!

4. Trying to Change Them. Like my daughter's first-grade teacher used to say, "You get what you get, and you don't throw a fit." If you genuinely like him or her, accept them as he is. Carmen lamented that she wished her date was more outgoing, but that's not something she can control. The only thing you can change is what he wears!

5. Trusting Too Fast. Trust takes time. On the first date, everyone puts their best foot forward. Observe their actions: Do they call when they say they will? Do they follow through on plans? Those behaviors build trust over time.

6. Too Many Drinks. If you're like Trina and get nervous on first dates, resist the urge to pregame with cocktails. Having three glasses of wine can lead to a sloppy evening. Guys, lay off too many scotches on the rock to soothe your nerves. Instead, boost your confidence by going on more first dates.

From First Date to Second... and Beyond

7. Inviting Him Over Too Soon. Inviting a date to your home for dinner on a second date can feel like too much, too soon—unless it's a party setting. Generally, save the intimate dinners for later in the relationship.

8. Not Being Positive. Negativity can be a major turn-off. Avoid bashing exes, complaining about the dating site, or criticizing the weather. Instead, focus on uplifting conversations.

9. Bonus Tip: **Be Gracious!** A simple "thank you" can go a long way and is a major turn-on.
Avoiding these common pitfalls can lead to more meaningful connections. Remember, dating is about enjoying the journey, not just reaching the destination!

Andrea McGinty

WORKSHEET #9—
Am I Positive?

GREEN symbolizes thoughtfulness and balance in **Gift Giving 411.** Thoughtful gift-giving can reflect your care and attention, creating a foundation for meaningful gestures.

chapter 8
Gift Giving 411

#94 Get to Know Your Dating Calendar

A question I often hear—whether at a cocktail party or from someone who's just browsed my website—is: *When's the best time to start dating? Should I go online now, or wait to meet people in person?*

Well, let me ask you this: Is there ever a perfect time to get pregnant? Or to book that month-long glamping trip in a luxury RV? My answer: Anytime is the right time! Quit waiting for some magical date on the calendar—it doesn't exist. The only thing you're doing by waiting is getting one day older.

But after 30 years of experience in the dating world, both offline and online, I have noticed some quirks in seasonal dating patterns. Here's a month-by-month breakdown to give you some insight.

Gift Giving 411

January: New Year, New Love?

Absolutely! The New Year brings a surge of singles flocking to dating sites, eager to make their top resolution—finding love—come true. From the chilly streets of Caspar, Wyoming, to the sun-soaked beaches of San Diego, people are logging in, ready for a fresh start. While it's not a mass exodus to online dating, you will notice a fresh batch of profiles spurred on by that New Year's commitment.

February: Love is in the Air

Valentine's Day adds extra pressure, and yes, it works. The cold weather in much of the country doesn't deter singles from turning up the heat online. It's a busy month for dating, whether you love or loathe the Valentine's hype.

March, April, May: Spring Fever

As winter coats come off and spring wardrobes debut, so does the energy for dating. This is a time when optimism blooms alongside the flowers—making it a great time to dive into dating. Just remember, I recommend committing to dating for at least three months. Find a friend or support person to keep you motivated and grounded during this journey.

Andrea McGinty

Summer: Sun, Fun, and Romance

Some might wonder, "Isn't everyone on vacation?" Nope! We don't all live in Italy, where the entire country shuts down for a month. Summer is actually a fantastic time for dating—think outdoor concerts, farmer's markets, and street fairs. It's a playful season full of opportunities to meet people in fun, relaxed settings.

September-October: Back-to-School Vibes

There's a mini surge in dating activity that mirrors the excitement of back-to-school season. It's that feeling of starting something new as the crisp autumn air settles in. People are refreshed after summer and ready to refocus on finding a relationship. My mind is already racing ahead to where I want to be personally by the holidays.

November-December: Holiday Pressure and 'Cuffing Season'

The holiday season kicks into gear, and early November sees a spike in dating before Thanksgiving. There's often pressure to bring someone home for the holidays, or at least to avoid those awkward family questions about your love life. And yes, this also marks the start of "Cuffing Season"—a supposed time when people look for short-term relationships to get them through the colder months.

Do I believe in Cuffing Season? Not really. It's a catchy term, but I haven't seen much evidence of it, especially for singles in the 35-65 age group. So, don't stress over it or buy into the hype.

So, When's the Best Time to Date?

The answer isn't tied to any particular month or season, and it definitely isn't "when I lose 10 pounds on Ozempic." The best time to start dating is **today**! Stop waiting for the stars to align or the perfect moment to arrive. Your moment is now.

#95 The Ins And Out On Gift Giving

**The Joy of Giving:
Creating Memorable Moments**

Let's face it—everyone loves a good gift! Some people get excited about finding the perfect gift for someone else, while others just enjoy receiving them. Personally? I'm all about the giving. There's something magical about surprising someone and watching their face light up with joy, shock, or excitement. My favorite gifts to give? Experiences—hands down!

Looking back on some of my most memorable relationships, I can't help but smile at the experiences I've gifted. Once, I gave a boyfriend who loved fast cars a one-day racing course (nothing fancy like a Porsche—just pure speed and adrenaline).

Andrea McGinty

Another time, I booked a private spelunking tour through Kentucky caves for the two of us—yes, I was in on that adventure, too! For a new guy I was seeing, I opted for something low-key but fun—a cooking class at Sur La Table. We'd only been dating two months, so it wasn't over-the-top, but we had a blast making soufflés. Oh, and for our six-month anniversary, a couple's massage. He loved it. Now that I think about it, it seems I've been gifting myself a little bit with these experiences, too!

But why is gift-giving so important in relationships? Let's dig into why it matters—and how it can deepen intimacy, strengthen bonds, and keep the excitement alive.

#96 Thoughtfulness Speaks Volumes

Gifts are a tangible way of saying, "I thought about you." When you take time to choose something meaningful, it shows that you value your partner. And no, this doesn't mean you need to buy something every week. It's about occasional thoughtful gestures that remind your partner how much they mean to you.

Gift Giving 411

Why Gift-Giving Matters in Love

1. Actions Speak When Words Can't: Sometimes, people struggle to express their feelings verbally. Gifts can bridge that gap. One weekly "gift" I treasure? Jeff fills my car with gas, takes it to the car wash, and vacuums out all the dog hair left by my Golden Retriever, Luna. It's not flashy, but it's thoughtful—and I appreciate it more than words can say.

2. Creating Lasting Memories: Some gifts live on long after they're unwrapped. On my desk sits a bobblehead of my favorite Red Sox player, Triston Casas. It came with tickets to a Red Sox vs. Yankees game—talk about an unforgettable experience. And yes, while jewelry is nice, I'm all about the memories tied to a unique experience.

3. It's Romantic: Let's not forget—gift-giving is inherently romantic. Whether you've been with someone for a month or eight years, you need to nurture that intimacy. Thoughtful gifts help keep that connection alive. Relationships are special—they deserve a little watering now and then to help them grow.

Andrea McGinty

#97 The Big Gift-Giving Days... Valentine's

Ugh. I'm not a huge fan of the commercial pressure of Valentine's Day. What does Saint Valentine really have to do with lovers, anyway? Here's my history lesson of the day.

The Origin of Valentine's Day: A Brief History Lesson

Saint Valentine was a priest in Rome during the reign of Emperor Claudius II in the 3rd century AD, a time when the emperor banned marriages for young men, believing single men made better soldiers. Defying this decree, Valentine secretly performed marriages for young couples, which ultimately led to his arrest and imprisonment. While in jail, he reportedly healed the jailer's blind daughter, and before his execution, he sent her a note signed "Your Valentine," which is believed to have inspired the modern phrase used on Valentine's Day cards. Martyred around 269 AD, his feast day is celebrated on February 14, a date that has become associated with romantic love, particularly during the Middle Ages. It doesn't really make sense… but okay. So, back to regular programming.

Gift Giving 411

Three Months in? Communicate!

If dating for under one month, skip it. After a month or two, a card with a handwritten note will do. Avoid overspending on flowers or those over-the-top prix-fixe dinners. If you're three months in and exclusive, talk it out and see if you both feel the pressure—or agree to skip it altogether. But be sure to have that conversation so that one person doesn't show up with the goods, while the other does not. Awkward! Alternatively, consider volunteering together to spread the love in a meaningful way.

(Some people even break up before Valentine's Day just to avoid the pressure, so don't overthink it! Oh, and don't ever go on a first date on Valentine's Day!)

#98 Don't Let Valentine's Day Derail You

The *Love Actually* Perspective: More Than Just Romance

As Valentine's Day approaches, the questions begin: "What should I get him/her for a gift?" or "Andrea, do you think I'll have a date on Valentine's Day?" February 14th can evoke a mix of excitement and anxiety, whether you're in a relationship or not.

This holiday always makes me think of the movie *Love Actually* and all the different kinds of love we experience—romantic, unrequited, familial, cross-cultural, and even love that endures beyond death. There's so much more to love than just the romantic kind!

Single on February 14? No Problem

If you find yourself without a date this Valentine's Day, don't fret. First or second dates can be awkward and stressful, especially with the media hype surrounding the day. Unless you're in a committed relationship, a Valentine's date can often feel uncomfortable.

Remember, Valentine's Day is largely a Hallmark holiday designed to boost sales during a traditionally slow retail month. Think about it: candy, flowers (I heard from a friend at UPS about planes packed with flowers flown in from South America just for February 14), perfume, and all things pink and red.

Manage the Anxiety and Enjoy Cupid's Day

As a top dating coach, I often hear clients express their anxiety about this day—even weeks in advance! So, here's how to make the most of Cupid's Day without letting it stress you out:

1. Do Something Your Ex Hated: Order that Indian food she always complained about!

2. Take the Love Language Quiz: It's free and fun, plus it'll help you understand some of the profiles you see online.

Gift Giving 411

3. Explore Volunteer Opportunities: Consider giving back and making a positive impact in your community.

4. Indulge in Retail Therapy: Visit the cosmetics counter at Nordstrom and treat yourself to something new. Guys, maybe it's time for a new fragrance?

5. Plan a Trip: Research that getaway you've been dreaming about since COVID-19 hit.

6. Pamper Yourself: Book a facial and feel rejuvenated!

7. Create an Herb Window Box: Plant mint, basil, and thyme for fresh muddled cocktails at home.

8. Repair a Rift: Reach out to a loved one and mend any lingering issues. Remember that silly argument you had with your brother? Tell him you love him!

9. Bake Something Sweet: Surprise your awesome neighbor with homemade goodies—or grab some Girl Scout cookies!

10. Get Moving: Work out to a new cardio playlist. Those endorphins will lift your spirits!

Andrea McGinty

Valentine's Day is just one day out of 365—a day to celebrate all kinds of love, not just the romantic. We all love someone, so take a moment to reach out. On this day, I typically call my favorite aunt, who recently lost her husband. While I think of her often, I want to make sure we have a good long chat.

#99 Birthdays: A Day To Celebrate

Celebrating Birthdays: Knowing Your Partner's Preference

Birthdays should be celebrated, no matter the age. But keep in mind that some people aren't into the whole "birthday spectacle." My ex-husband hated birthday fuss, so we kept it simple with a homemade cake. Tailor your gift-giving to the person you're with, not what you think a birthday should be. If you've been dating for at least a month and have had a handful of dates, a book or something related to their interests is a good start. After three months? Think event tickets or something fun and interactive.

Gift Giving 411

**Thoughtful Gifts:
Matching the Stage of Your Relationship**

1. Less than 1 month: A card is perfect.

2. Dating for 1 month (and you've been on at least 4-5 dates): Consider a thoughtful book on a topic they're interested in, or something simple like a new dog collar or leash for their pet.

3. 3 months and exclusive: Step it up with sporting event tickets, concert or theater tickets, a nice dinner, Apple AirPods, or a tech gadget.

4. 6 months and exclusive: You can go for a weekend getaway, a necklace, or a bigger tech item like an iPad. Keep your budget in mind–this could range from $100 to $1000 depending on your situation.

(Avoid generic gift cards unless it's for a luxurious spa day at a specific spa. No $150 catch-all cards.)

#100 Anniversaries: Keep It In Perspective

Keep Perspective on the Timeline

Anniversaries are important but be mindful of the timeline. Throwing a surprise party for a two-month anniversary? You might not see them again! Keep it thoughtful but proportionate to the amount of time you've been together.

#101 Just-Because Gifts

Thoughtful Gestures Over Grand Presents

These might be my favorite. A small, thoughtful gift—like the six tiny sterling spoons I brought back for a guy who loved making charcuterie boards—can mean more than something extravagant. Once, a client of mine brought his girlfriend of three months a Turkish robe from a trip. She loved it—and now they're married! Sometimes, the smallest gestures leave the biggest impact.

Gift Giving 411

#102 *Rules Of Thumb*

Guidelines for Navigating Gift-Giving in Early Relationships

These aren't written in stone but are a solid guideline when treading into uncertain terrain.

1. Too much, too soon can be overwhelming and scare a lover away. Don't go overboard early on.

2. Holiday Gifting: Keep It Flexible! When it comes to the major holidays—Christmas, Hanukkah, Kwanzaa—remember, not everyone is in a "Hallmark movie" mood. Some people struggle during this time of year. But if your partner is the festive type, plan something that suits both of you. It could be as simple as attending a town event like a tree lighting, or something more personal like cooking a holiday meal together. My favorite holiday tradition? Each year, we pick a country (last year it was Lebanon, this year it's France), and we prepare a special meal with friends and family. It's an experience we cherish—and talk about for months beforehand.

3. The Bottom Line: Experiences Matter! Gifts can range from luxurious items like lingerie or an alma mater scarf to grand gestures like a ski trip or a day volunteering together. But the most meaningful gifts are shared experiences. At the end of the day, gift-giving in relationships doesn't have to be about flashy items or big price tags. What really matters is the thought and the time you spend together. Experiences, in particular, have a way of fostering intimacy and building memories that last far longer than any material gift. So, the next time you're thinking about what to give, think beyond the wrapping paper and go for something that will bring you closer together. Back to the experiential gifts!

#103 Prepare Yourself For Summer Love

Summer Dating Tips for the Season Ahead

With Memorial Day just around the corner, dating apps and websites are buzzing with activity. The warmer weather and increased social interactions make it an ideal time to connect with someone special. Here are some tips to help you maximize your summer dating experience:

Gift Giving 411

1. Embrace the Natural Look: While personal style is subjective, consider opting for a more relaxed and natural look during the summer. This might mean ditching the heavy makeup or opting for a lighter beard style. Remember, confidence is key, and feeling comfortable in your own skin is attractive.

2. Prioritize Safety: Summer dating should be fun, but it's essential to prioritize your safety. If concerned, consider taking a self-defense class or refreshing your safety skills. Personally, I think everyone should take a self-defense class once in their life! This can boost your confidence and help you feel more secure in any situation, but when it comes to the online dating world, I am 99.9% sure you will be just fine using common sense. Remember, meet at a safe neutral location such as a restaurant or wine bar for the first date!

3. Update Your Profile: Your dating profile is your first impression. Ensure your photos are current, well-lit, and showcase your personality. Regularly update your bio to reflect your current interests and goals. A stale profile can deter potential matches.

4. Be Proactive and Efficient: Don't let conversations linger online for too long. Aim to meet potential matches within a reasonable timeframe. If you've been chatting for weeks without making plans, it might be time to move on.

5. Refresh Your Wardrobe: A fresh wardrobe can boost your confidence and make you feel more attractive. Invest in a few summer essentials that suit your style. Don't be afraid to experiment with new trends or colors.

6. Develop a Strategy: Approach dating with a plan. Set goals, such as how many matches you'll aim to make each week or how often you'll go on dates. Actively engage with the dating platform, send thoughtful messages, and be open to new connections.

7. Be yourself: Authenticity is attractive. Don't try to be someone you're not.

8. Have fun: Dating should be enjoyable. Don't put too much pressure on yourself.

9. Be respectful: Treat everyone with kindness and respect, regardless of the outcome.

Gift Giving 411

#104 Unwrap The Holidays With Ease

**Holiday Romance:
Embracing the Festive Spirit**

Tis the season! The holiday season is a wonderful time to connect with others and find love. Despite the hustle and bustle, many singles are open to dating and enjoying the festive atmosphere. Here are some tips to help you navigate the holiday dating scene:

1. Embrace the Season: Don't let the holiday rush deter you from dating. Attend festive events, parties, and gatherings. You never know who you might meet. Remember, the holiday spirit can be contagious, so embrace the joy and excitement of the season.

2. Gift Giving: When it comes to gifts, keep it thoughtful and appropriate for the stage of your relationship. Consider their interests and hobbies. As I mentioned above, experiences and more experiences! But if you are looking for a little something, here are a few more gift ideas:

- **For the Book lover:** A classic novel or a cozy blanket to enjoy while reading

- **For the sports fanatic:** Tickets to a game or merchandise from their favorite team

- **For the yogi:** A yoga mat or meditation accessories.

- **For the music lover:** Tickets to a concert or a curated playlist.

3. Be Understanding of Time Constraints: During the holidays, people may be busier than usual due to family visits, work commitments, and social events. Be understanding if they don't respond immediately to your messages. It doesn't necessarily mean they're losing interest.

4. Take It Slow: Avoid rushing into serious commitments too quickly. Getting to know someone takes time, and the holidays can be a whirlwind of activity. Enjoy the dating process and let the relationship develop naturally.

5. Embrace the Festive Spirit: Have fun and enjoy the holiday festivities together. Whether it's ice skating, baking cookies, or attending a Christmas market, creating shared experiences can strengthen your connection. Don't be afraid to try new things and embrace your inner child.

Gift Giving 411

#105 Navigating The "New" in The Holiday Era

**Keeping It Cool:
Managing the Festive Rush**

A new lover? Not quite exclusive? Getting serious but it is all still a little fresh and not quite sure if family and colleague intros are on the cards? Don't sweat it; I've got some words of wisdom about how to handle the Holiday bombardment while still treading the early relationship phase.

1. Communicate Your Expectations: If you have specific holiday plans or expectations, be open and honest with your potential partner. Clear communication can help prevent misunderstandings and ensure that both of you are on the same page.

2. Avoid Rushing: While it's tempting to accelerate a relationship during the holidays, it's important to take things at your own pace. A healthy relationship will withstand the test of time, so don't feel pressured to move too quickly.

3. Choose a Non-Holiday Date: Avoid scheduling your first date on a major holiday like New Year's Eve. This can create unnecessary pressure and expectations. Go for a more casual setting where you can get to know each other without the added stress of a holiday celebration.

4. Attend a Social Event Together: Once you've been on a few dates, consider attending a holiday party or social event together. This can provide valuable insights into their personality, social skills, and how they interact with others.

5. Don't Feel Pressured to Be a Plus-One: If you're not ready to meet their family or friends during the early stages of dating, it's perfectly acceptable to decline invitations to holiday gatherings. It's a sign of respect for your feelings and the pace of the relationship.

6. Give Each Other Space: Remember that your partner may have existing holiday plans or commitments. Respect their need for space and time with loved ones. It's important to maintain a balance between spending time together and honoring your individual lives.

7. Enjoy the Experience: The holiday season offers a unique opportunity to connect with someone special. Embrace the festive atmosphere, have fun, and enjoy the process of getting to know your potential partner.

Gift Giving 411

#106 Launch into the New Year with a Dating Bang

**Skip the Resolutions:
Build Real Dating Habits**

Since 75% of New Year's resolutions fail by the end of January, let's skip them for your love life this year! Sure, committing to a pricey gym membership might keep you motivated, but without accountability, most plans fall apart. Instead, let's dive into some practical 2023 dating tips from your dating coach! (By the way, January and February are peak months for online dating—singles across the country flock to dating apps, no matter the weather. Stats from Gallup and Pew prove it!)

New Year Dating Tips

1. Think outside your "type." You may always go for the 6'2" athlete or the 5'9" blonde, but love can surprise you. I've seen many people fall for someone they swore wasn't their type.

2. Don't expect perfection. And don't expect it from yourself either! Embrace imperfections.

3. Your date is not a mind reader. A healthy relationship needs communication, chemistry, and shared values. Did I mention communication?

4. Trust your gut. If something feels off—like a sketchy profile or one suspicious photo—listen to your instincts.

5. Don't get attached too quickly. One date doesn't mean "the one." Rushing to quit dating others after one great date? Bad idea.

6. Dive into online dating. Set a goal for 5 first dates in the first two weeks. It'll build your confidence, especially if you've been out of the dating scene for a while.

7. Say "Yes." Whether it's a party, a hike with new people, or a date with someone you're unsure about, take the chance. You never know where it might lead.

8. Live in the moment. Stop worrying about date #3 or how it will work with your kids. Focus on enjoying the present moment.

9. Don't overthink if they stop texting. If they ghost you, don't dwell on it. There's a huge dating pool out there—move on!

10. Know what you deserve. Never settle. In my 25 years as a dating coach, I've learned one thing: there's a lid for every pot, and I see it happen every day!

Gift Giving 411

11. High-Yield Tasks. Elon Musk uses the Pareto Principle to focus on the 20% of tasks that deliver 80% of the results. I teach my clients to do the same: maximize your time on dating apps by working smarter, not harder.

12. Half In/Half Out. If you're not fully committed to dating, don't waste your time—or your money with me.

13. Get Off the Fence. It's time to make a decision to go for it. Sitting on the fence only gives you a sore butt.

14. Look in the Mirror. Not for a Botox check! Your dating success starts with you. While I can guide you, your attitude is key to ending up in my 65% success rate.

15. Share Your Goals. Sharing your goals makes you accountable. Richard Branson swears by this, and just look at all he's accomplished while having fun!

16. Surround Yourself with Smart, Positive People. This one's simple: positivity is contagious.

17. Lunch with a Friend Weekly. My mom always told me to have lunch with a friend each week, even with six kids in the house. It keeps you fresh, interesting, and happy—and happy people make great dates.

18. Be More Interesting. We all have 1440 minutes in a day—it's how you use them that counts. Want to be up to date on fascinating topics? Try reading 1440 News. It only takes a few minutes, and it's a great way to stay informed. Better yet, it's free online and I am a big fan!

19. Self-Confidence Gets You Everywhere. As Ken Jennings of *Jeopardy* fame says, "Self-esteem is important because it sets up a powerful cycle of self-growth and risk-taking." Confidence is attractive—and it can take you places.

20. Don't Let Information Overwhelm You. Limit your media and social media consumption. Too much information can cloud your mind and keep you from focusing on what really matters.

While I'm not big on New Year's resolutions, the start of a new year does bring fresh opportunities. So, here's to a fresh go around the sun—let's make it your best dating year yet!

#107 Get Your New Year's Dating Mind Right

When my clients find themselves in a funk heading into the bang of a clock reset, I remind them of these nuggets to lift them up and out. Pick your favorite and write it out in the space below until it worms its way into your psyche and hangs out there. (Feel free to do more than one or write out your own!)

Gift Giving 411

Positive Reminders to Kickstart the New Year

1. "Plant seeds every single day that you know who you are, you know what you're about and you know what goals you've set for yourself." — **Stephen Curry** As a Steph Curry fan, I love how he simplifies growth. One seed a day? We all have time for that. In dating, it's like sending one unique message a day to someone who sparks your interest.

2. "I don't know where I'm going from here, but I promise it won't be boring." — **David Bowie** When it comes to online dating, Bowie's right. First dates can lead to anything—boring is not on the menu!

3. "Life is short" really means 'do something.'" — **Chimamanda Adichie** No room for procrastination here—dive into the dating pool and take action!

4. "They always say time changes things, but you have to change them yourself." — **Andy Warhol** Singles who take proactive and creative approaches to dating find success. Don't wait for someone to knock on your door—go out and make things happen.

5. "Age is not the enemy. Stagnation and complacency are the enemies." — **Twyla Tharp**

Andrea McGinty

In over 25 years as a dating coach, I've seen age matter less and less. Today, singles in their 40s to 70s are more active and vibrant than ever. Don't let age or complacency stop you—get out there!

I had one client in Kansas City, Lynn, who at 58 was ready to give up after 14 first dates. I encouraged her to give Henry, 54, a shot. Today, they're sending me holiday cards of their blended family at the Rockefeller skating rink—success stories like this are why I love what I do!

WORKSHEET #10—
Favorite Life or Dating Quotes

TEAL signifies calmness and balance, when **Dealing with Setbacks and Negativity,** which is helpful for managing negative experiences and staying centered in dating.

chapter 9
Dealing with Setbacks and Negativity

#108 Handling Rejection and Moving Forward

**Rejection Isn't the End:
Navigating Setbacks with Confidence**

Your first date isn't up for a second? Or did things fall apart after several dates? Don't sweat it. I understand that rejection is a tough pill to swallow, but it's a normal part of the dating forum. Nobody out there has a perfect score.

Nevertheless, it is easy to take things personally, especially when you're not getting the desired results. Remember, it's a numbers game. Everyone experiences setbacks, but you have to stay in the game.

Dealing with Setbacks and Negativity

I had a rough patch once when a guy, Jack, I really liked. Jack insisted I keep the Fourth of July free so he could take me to the fireworks and some "great" events—but then acted like a confused deer in the headlights when I asked a couple of days in advance what we were doing. Jack proceeded to shrug and say he was going to stay in. What the?

We had *had* several amazing dates before this, so this nonchalant attitude came out of left field. It stung, but I realized it wasn't about me but about him being a jerk. It's about maintaining perspective and not letting one person's actions define your dating experience.

It's okay to feel disappointed but don't let it consume you. Keep putting yourself out there; eventually, you'll find someone who appreciates you. I will keep reiterating that dating, just like this book, is a numbers game. Eventually you will draw a winner.

#109 Treasure Your Support System

**Stay Grounded:
Cultivating Your Support System**

Having a dedicated support system and maintaining your own life is pivotal when navigating the ups and downs of dating.

Whether you're riding high on the thrill of a new connection or weathering the storm of rejection, having friends to confide in can make all the difference. Continue nurturing your friendships, hobbies, and personal interests. This not only enriches your life but also prevents your relationship from becoming the sole focus.

Sure, it is tempting to become completely absorbed in a new relationship, but maintaining your independence and existing friendships is equally important. A healthy relationship is built on two strong individuals, not one person sacrificing their entire life for another. So, keep those social connections alive, and cherish the support and laughter they bring to your life.

**Maintain Your Identity:
The Key to Healthy Relationships**

We also don't want you to lose you in this process. Preserve your individuality while building a robust connection. If you loved pottery or squash or fencing before—don't stop. A healthy partnership thrives when both individuals have fulfilling lives outside of the relationship.

Conversely, neglecting your social circle and personal growth can strain a relationship. It's important to maintain balance and avoid becoming overly dependent on your partner.

Dealing with Setbacks and Negativity

#110 Maintain An Upbeat Attitude

I know all too well that online dating can be overwhelming, but with the right mindset and strategies, it can be a rewarding experience. Here are some key points to remind yourself:

1. Maintain a Positive Outlook. Focus on the possibilities rather than dwelling on setbacks. It only takes one connection to be effective.

2. Set Realistic Expectations. Avoid putting immense pressure on every date. Enjoy the process of getting to know someone new without expecting perfection.

3. Take Breaks. Online dating can be exhausting. It's okay to step back and recharge.

4. Expand Your Horizons. Try new activities and meet new people to keep things fresh and exciting.

5. Trust Your Instincts. If something feels off, it probably is. Don't ignore your gut feelings.

6. Be Patient. Finding the right person takes time. Don't rush the process.

Dating is about discovering compatibility and building connections. By staying positive and open-minded, you increase your chances of finding a fulfilling relationship.

I encourage you to examine the questions below and write down your answers. You can return to this whenever necessary throughout your dating quest—it is a good gauge of where your mind is at and the holes that might need stitching.

Time to fill out the worksheet!

#111 Phrases Confident Singles Use

Overcoming Negative Thoughts: The Battle Within

Yes, how you self-talk creates your success… or failure. In life. In dating. In everything, right?

Quick example: I have a new 56-year-old client who told me she wasn't sure anyone would want to date her—after all, she was widowed. I'm looking at her on our Zoom call thinking, "What? She's darling! Dimples, gracious Texan accent, and in great shape."

And I said, directly and bluntly, don't ever say or think that again. Otherwise, she was quite confident on the call—just married so long and nervous about her very first date. Science has proven we have something like 80,000 thoughts a day—and 60-70% are negative. OMG! Startling. And no, I have absolutely no idea how someone figured that out.

Dealing with Setbacks and Negativity

WORKSHEET #11— My Attitude Questionnaire

Creating Affirmative Mantras

Upward and onward on how you should be talking to yourself:

1. I make my own decisions, take the actions, and am responsible for the results. You betcha. So, last week you played a lot of golf or tennis, binged on the latest Netflix series, and went online once for 20 minutes. You now have no dates this week. Decision + Actions = No Dates.

2. My past needn't be my future. Sure, the past shapes us and has an enormous impact on who we are today. Is change possible? My mom (thinking of you, Mom, as I write this) once told me the only certainty in life is change. She wasn't talking about dating, just life in general. You may have been in an unhappy marriage. You may feel you wasted five years on a man who couldn't commit. Intelligent people learn from these mistakes. And guess what? When I'm working with them, they see red flags after 1, 2, or maybe 3 dates and cut it off immediately. The past did affect the future in a fantastic way in dates!

3. I'm not easily influenced by others' opinions. I can't stress this one enough! How many clients have told me horror stories their friends have shared about online dating? Tons. I always laugh. Oh my gosh, this isn't 2005 or 2010 when the online dating sphere was still figuring out safety features. How about this one: "My married friends tell me online dating is for losers." And your married friends' solution is…? And they know this how?

4. Self-care is not the same as selfishness. If you're not taking care of yourself, who will?

5. Optimism leads to achievement. If you think you are going to meet someone, you will. If you don't, you won't.

Dealing with Setbacks and Negativity

#112 How To Kick Your Dating Doubts To The Curb

Overcoming "Date" Anxiety
We all grapple with insecurities that can hinder our happiness and love lives. Overcoming these doubts is crucial to finding love. While it's impossible to feel confident all the time, recognizing and addressing these feelings is the first step.

To boost your confidence and overcome dating anxiety, try these tips:

1. Face your fears: Acknowledge your insecurities to begin overcoming them. Practice social interactions to build confidence in meeting new people.

2. Set realistic goals: Avoid putting unnecessary pressure on yourself. Focus on progress rather than perfection.

3. Learn from setbacks: View dating challenges as opportunities for growth. Don't let failures discourage you; focus on what you can learn.

4. Embrace your individuality: Accept your flaws and strengths. Celebrate your unique qualities.

5. Challenge negative thoughts: Recognize that negative thoughts are temporary. Practice mindfulness techniques to manage anxiety.

6. Surround yourself with positivity: Build a support system of encouraging friends who uplift you.

7. Learn from others: Seek inspiration from stories of people who've overcome similar challenges.

8. Prioritize self-care: Engage in activities that bring you joy and relaxation.

9. Let go of negativity: Distance yourself from people or situations that contribute to your insecurities.

10. Celebrate small victories: Acknowledge your progress and reward yourself for taking steps forward.

Finding love is an expedition. Be patient with yourself, focus on personal growth, and maintain a positive outlook.

Dealing with Setbacks and Negativity

#113 *How To Stay Positive When Dating Seems To Suck*

Online dating can be overwhelming and disheartening. It's common to feel exhausted, frustrated, or discouraged. However, remember that countless success stories emerge from the digital dating world.

Tips for Maintaining a Positive Outlook

To maintain a positive outlook:

1. Lower your expectations: Focus on enjoying the process rather than fixating on finding "the one."

2. Limit screen time: Dedicate specific, short periods to online dating to avoid burnout.

3. Take breaks: Step away from dating apps entirely for a fleeting period to recharge.

4. Explore new interests: Diversify your life with hobbies and activities to meet people organically.

5. Control what you can: Focus on being selective and setting boundaries.

6. Don't take rejection personally: Understand that dating involves trying and sometimes failing.

7. Maintain perspective: Dating is one part of your life, not your entire world.

8. Manage expectations: Avoid building unrealistic hopes based on limited information.

9. Date multiple people: Don't put all your eggs in one basket.

10. Stay persistent: Success often comes after overcoming challenges.

Countless individuals have found love through online dating. Stay positive, be patient, and enjoy the voyage—including the bumps and stormy seas that may come.

#114 Don't Slip Back into Divorce Regret

Trusting the Process

When the going gets tough with dating, as in life, it can be easy for some to slip back into divorce regret—dwelling on the notion that the grass isn't greener on the other side, wishing they had tried harder to make it work, and even tempted to text the ex and explore the options.

Remind yourself of the reason why it ended. Accept that what is done is done. Pull your shoulders back.

Give me a smile. You've embarked on this incredible new life chapter, and amazing things await.

It will happen. I can't wave a magic wand and tell you when. But on average, my clients fall into incredible, loving long-term relationships typically within three months to two years. Stay at it. You've got this.

Andrea McGinty

#115 Responding To Criticism From Loved Ones

The Evolving Perception of Online Dating

The stigma surrounding online dating has significantly diminished in recent years. While I've encountered some resistance, particularly from older generations, the overall attitude has shifted. It's important to manage expectations and be prepared for potential criticism. Emphasize the positives of online dating while acknowledging concerns.

Focusing on the present is crucial when addressing skepticism. Reassure loved ones that you're taking steps to ensure safety and are enjoying the process.

Dealing with Setbacks and Negativity

#116 Reasons Why It May Not Be Working For You-Yet

We've all heard the saying, "Can't see the forest for the trees." This often happens when we're too fixated on the details of a problem. Sometimes, an outsider's perspective is needed. Are you bombing online dating?

Five Signs Your Approach Might Be Off

1. Lack of First Dates: If you haven't been on at least four or five first dates in the past month, you're doing something wrong. Online dating is a tool, not a destination. Real connections happen in person.

2. Unrealistic Expectations: Believing every potential match must be nearly perfect on paper is setting yourself up for disappointment. While it's important to have standards, don't let perfectionism hold you back. Chemistry, communication, and shared values often emerge in person.

3. Free Dating Sites Only: You dipped a toe in it. Don't kid yourself-your heart and soul are not into dating. Using free dating platforms exclusively might be limiting your options. Investing in a paid subscription often provides access to a higher quality pool of potential matches.

4. Infrequent Logins: Checking your dating profiles once a week isn't enough. Online dating is competitive, and opportunities can disappear quickly. Consistent engagement is key. You know what will help you? Accountability! Yes, a dating coach (that's me!).

5. Making Excuses: Busy schedules, travel plans, or seasonal changes shouldn't derail your dating efforts. Successful people prioritize dating alongside other key areas of their lives. My guess is you don't ignore your children or workouts or golf...

Online dating is a numbers game! (Yes, I will keep drilling this into you!) Stay positive, be proactive, (I will keep on this one like a broken record, too) and don't hesitate to seek professional guidance if needed.

#117 Lessons Learned

There's no shortage of lessons to be learned in the domain of online dating. It's a blend of art, science, math and a bit of luck. Here are some insights gleaned from my clients:

Dealing with Setbacks and Negativity

Lesson 1: Quantity Leads to Quality

Many people feel discouraged early on. However, it often takes meeting several people before finding a great match. Carrie, a client of mine, experienced this firsthand. After 14 first dates in 3 months and feeling disheartened, she met James, and their connection was immediate. It's a reminder that persistence pays off.

Lesson 2: Less is More When Texting

Over-communication can hinder progress. Danny, another client, discovered that sending multiple messages to potential matches wasn't effective. Sometimes, less is more, allowing anticipation and interest to build.

Andrea McGinty

#118 Brutally Honest Reasons You're Still Single

Being single is a choice, whether conscious or not. While life gets busy, it's paramount to prioritize finding a partner if that's your goal. Unlike past generations, today's dating landscape offers unprecedented opportunities through online platforms. With millions of singles actively searching, there's no excuse not to take advantage of these resources.

Successful online dating requires dedication and a willingness to step outside your comfort zone.

5 Reasons You Might Still Be Single

1. Inertia: While you may express a desire for a relationship, consistent action is crucial. Proactivity is key to achieving your goals, just as it is in your career.

Dealing with Setbacks and Negativity

2. Negativity: A pessimistic outlook can hinder your dating success. Negative self-talk and generalizations about potential partners create self-fulfilling prophecies.

3. Rigid Expectations: Having overly specific criteria can limit your options. Flexibility and open-mindedness are necessary for finding compatibility.

4. Overeagerness: Coming on too strong can be a turn-off. A first date should be a casual and enjoyable experience, not an interrogation.

5. Giving Up Too Soon: Disappointing experiences can lead to discouragement. It's important to persist and learn from setbacks.

#119 A Roundup of Frequently Asked Questions

When to Start Dating Again?

Answer: There's no set time. It's about when you feel both nervous and excited. There's no perfect season to begin dating, just like there's no perfect time for other life events!

Dealing with Jealousy

Answer: Don't compare yourself to others. And don't compare your body to when you were 25 when you are now 55.

Why No Second Dates?

Answer: Review your first date behavior. Ask yourself if you were self-centered, too negative, or treated it like an interview. Seek feedback after several dates to identify patterns. I found this quite interesting—I have a client who's used my coaching services twice already. She's 66, attractive, living in Dallas, and has been on plenty of first dates but not many second ones.

Dealing with Setbacks and Negativity

Recently, she called me for another round of coaching, and I said, "Carol, let me think about this. Something's off. I don't want you to keep paying me without us figuring out what's going on—give me a week to do some due diligence."

Now, I really like Carol. She's a former New Yorker living in Texas, with a classic Type A personality—impatient, direct, a bit terse. A true CEO type, which I totally understand because I'm the same way.

So, I went back through every single match she had over the past two years (thankfully, I take copious notes!), and I started noticing a pattern—both in her initial texts and things she said on first dates. For example, on one date, she told a dentist, "You seem a little cheap." To a chiropractor she liked, she asked at the end of the first date, "Are you attracted to me?"

You can probably see where this was going. So, for round three, we focused on fixing her approach—not changing her personality but tweaking how she interacted. And did it work? Absolutely. I'm not sure who's happier—Carol or me!

Online Messaging Tips

Answer: For every 7 messages, expect 1 response. Keep your messages short, friendly, and fun. Avoid being too brief or writing long paragraphs.

Long-Distance Relationships—Yes or No?

Answer: Mostly no. Be realistic about your willingness to relocate if you're deeply connected to your current city.

When to Have Sex?

Answer: There are no rules. It's about when you feel comfortable. For some, it's casual, for others, it involves emotions. Do what feels right for you.

Sharing Personal Information

Answer: Avoid disclosing personal details like disabilities or family issues in your profile. Share this after a few dates once you've built a connection.

Dating Costs

Answer: Expect to pay $20-$50 per month on top dating sites and apps.

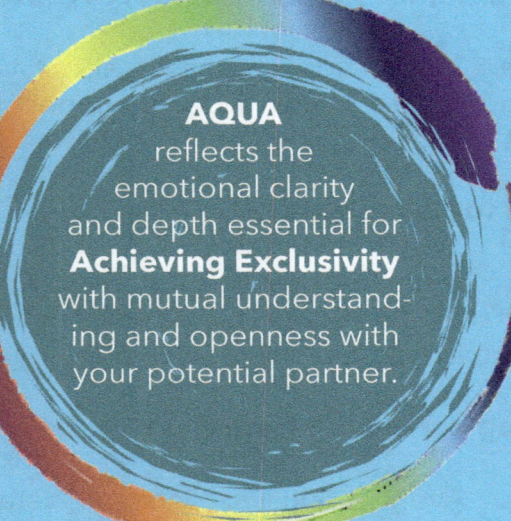

AQUA
reflects the emotional clarity and depth essential for **Achieving Exclusivity** with mutual understanding and openness with your potential partner.

chapter 10
Achieving Exclusivity

#120 Having The "Exclusive" Conversation

So, you've been seeing someone for a few months, or a few weeks if the flames are on fire, and the question of exclusivity inevitably arises. This is where the art of conversation is critical. I'm not a fan of "you just know." Nope, you don't.

**Exclusivity:
Finding the Right Moment and Words**

Exclusivity is pretty important, to put it mildly—important enough that it should be articulated. However, this should arise at a time when you feel you have both naturally reached this point and feel comfortable having what can be a fairly uncomfortable conversation. There's no strict timeline, yet open communication is key. It's not about ultimatums or grand gestures; it's about expressing your feelings and ascertaining where the other person is at.

Achieving Exclusivity

It need not be a super serious sit-down discussion, but rather a casual conversation about your expectations that can clear the air and prevent misunderstandings. Perhaps you are watching Sunday football together and you can casually comment, "I think I am going to delete my dating apps; I don't want to date other people."

Building Trust Through Communication

Another approach?
Playfully ask: "Do you like me? Or do you like, *like* me—as in, you don't like like anyone else?" And let things roll from there.
Exclusivity is a two-way street. Both partners should feel at ease and secure in the relationship. If you're sensing hesitation or inconsistency when you mention this, it might be time for a more direct conversation on what you want. Ultimately, the goal with this conversation is to build a foundation of trust and respect, and that starts with honest communication.
Just because someone is seeing you exclusively doesn't guarantee a happily ever after. Savor the journey and don't put too much pressure on yourself or your partner.

Andrea McGinty

#121 To Bed and When To Bed

Dating and Intimacy Over 45: A New Perspective

When it comes to dating in the 45-50 and over age group, the dynamics of relationships are different from what many may have experienced in their 20s and 30s. Most people in this stage of life are seeking long-term relationships with the player days long in the rearview mirror. Subsequently, the approach to dating—and especially to physical intimacy—reflects that shift. Women, in particular, often feel that they cannot or do not want to sleep with multiple partners at the same time, due to the emotional and physical demands involved. Some may call that stereotyping, but I just call it the reality. Stereotypes exist for a reason.

On the other hand, some men may still approach dating with a more casual mindset initially, as seen in the example of an engineer client, Adam, who dated multiple women after his long-term marriage ended before eventually settling into an exclusive relationship. Adam needed that hedonistic window to reach a place of calm and readiness. The timeline for when to become intimate varies widely from person to person and situation to situation.

Timing Intimacy:
There Are No Hard and Fast Rules

There are no strict rules about when it's the "right" time to sleep with someone. The idea of rigid guidelines, like those presented in the book *The Rules* from the late 90s, is largely outdated. Instead, it's about feeling ready and ensuring the circumstances are right—whether that means waiting for an emotional connection to develop or simply taking advantage of the opportunity when it arises. I've had friends and clients sleep with their date on the first night, and I've had others wait weeks, or even months, to consummate the relationship. Some have gone on to have long and fulfilling relationships and marriages, and others have fizzled out, irrespective of the bed clock variable.

Sex remains an important and enjoyable part of life for many, even into their 60s and 70s, reflecting a broader cultural shift from past generations where it might have been less openly acknowledged. Whether you're a man or a woman, the key is to listen to your own feelings and needs and proceed when it feels right for you.

Andrea McGinty

#122 Take Care of the Buzz Kills

Navigating Intimacy Challenges for Women Over 50

As people navigate dating in their 50s and beyond, they often encounter unique challenges related to intimacy that weren't as prevalent in their younger years. For women, menopause can bring about a decrease in libido and issues such as dryness, which can make sexual activity less comfortable. Hormone replacement therapy (HRT) can be a game-changer, helping to restore libido and alleviate dryness, and other women have found success with naturopathic remedies. This is very individual; but I urge you not to sit idly and let "nature take its toll." There is a breadth of knowledge and options out there for women now, and we owe it to our ancestors to go for it! In any case, it is important for women to be proactive by consulting with their gynecologist before jumping back into the dating pool, ensuring that any potential issues are addressed early on.

Achieving Exclusivity

Men's Challenges and the Importance of Proactivity

Men, too, face their own set of challenges as they age, particularly around maintaining sexual performance. (I strongly advise you to check in with your doctor, too!) Factors like being overweight, drinking alcohol, and smoking can exacerbate these issues, leading to difficulties in achieving and maintaining an erection.

For both men and women, patience is a cornerstone. It's natural for intimacy to require a bit more effort and understanding at this stage in life, and rushing or pressuring oneself or a partner can make the experience more stressful and less enjoyable.

Patience, Communication, and Embracing Change

Also, keep in mind that the ability to achieve orgasm may change with age. Women in their 50s and 60s might find that reaching orgasm is less frequent compared to when they were younger. This is completely normal, and it's important not to put undue pressure on oneself. Open communication with a gynecologist—and our partners—can also provide valuable advice and strategies to navigate these changes, helping to maintain a satisfying and enjoyable sex life.

Andrea McGinty

#123 Not So Taboo Topics... like STDs

Prioritizing Sexual Health: An Essential Conversation

It's surprising how few people openly discuss STDs these days. Growing up in a time when the topic was taboo, I expected this factor to be a constant concern, especially for the young who talk much more freely about their sexual exploits than older generations. However, it seems that younger generations are actually more relaxed about it. That said, prioritize sexual health.

Safety First: Know Your Status

If you're dating someone with a history of multiple partners, regardless of their age, asking for an STD test is completely reasonable. After all, condoms aren't foolproof, and everyone deserves to know their status. Plus, let's face it, sex is often more enjoyable without one. Health first! Get it over with early in the game, and you're free to have some fun without the anxiety!

#124 Getting Down With the Sexy Stuff

**Embracing Confidence:
Refresh Your Lingerie Wardrobe**

Age is no barrier with regards to feeling sexy and confident. A great starting point? Ladies let's start with lingerie. After years in the same relationship or marriage, it's common for lingerie to become an afterthought. Many women might find their underwear drawer full of old, worn-out items that no longer make them feel attractive. Taking the time to refresh your collection with beautiful, well-fitting pieces can do wonders for your self-esteem. Visiting a store like Nordstrom or Neiman Marcus, where staff are trained to properly fit bras, can be an eye-opening experience. Many (some studies say up to 80%) of women don't realize they're wearing the wrong size which can affect both comfort and appearance. A well-fitted bra, no matter the size, can look incredibly sexy and boost confidence.

Sleepwear Makeover: Elevate Your Comfort and Style

Updating your sleepwear is another uncomplicated way to enhance your sense of sensuality. If you've been sleeping in oversized t-shirts or old pajamas, consider treating yourself to something more flattering and fun. Cute, comfortable sleepwear can make you feel better about yourself, even when you're just lounging at home. And don't forget about the importance of sexy underwear—whether you're single or in a relationship, wearing something that makes you feel good can have a positive impact on your mood and confidence.

#125 Open To Experimentation

What is great about reaching the second half of life and embarking on a new lease of the dating days? There is a sense of liberation many of us may not have experienced in our younger years.

A New Chapter:
Embracing Liberation in the Second Half of Life

As people enter a new phase of life after a long-term marriage, particularly one that might have been more traditional or "vanilla," there's often a desire to explore and embrace newfound sexual freedom. After years in a conventional relationship, the prospect of experimenting with new experiences—such as threesomes or other forms of sexual exploration—can feel like an exciting new chapter.
This openness is especially true for those in their late 40s to 60s, who may have had limited exposure to diverse sexual experiences when they were younger due to the lack of resources like the internet or the availability of different perspectives on sexuality. For those who haven't been sexually active in a while, it's perfectly okay to explore sex toys. Adding a few items to your collection can help reignite your sexual energy and make solo or partnered play more enjoyable. Many stores offer a wide range of options, from lubricants to vibrators, and the staff at these shops are usually knowledgeable and non-judgmental. Don't be afraid to ask for   recommendations or advice—they're there to help you find what works best for you. I like the stores best; versus online. The staff can explain what it does and if you're nervous, go when the store opens and not at 11pm at night. These stores have loooong hours! Taking the time to explore your desires and preferences is a healthy and empowering step in embracing your sexuality.

Ok, this book is personal to me. Very. So after my marriage, I had not been "intimate" in 4 years. Was I nervous about having sex? You bet. So, here we go: one morning around 10 am I passed by an inviting Sexxy Shoppe in Delray Beach and saw no cars in the parking lot. Yay. (By the way, it looked "classy", not sordid if that's what you are imagining.) I went in and I had so much fun and learned so much in an hour as their only customer. What a knowledgeable and easy to talk with staff. From the best lube to……, ok, that's a bit too personal. Suffice to say I walked out happy, excited and confident to try some new things.

**Redefining Sexuality:
Confidence and Exploration After 50**

Today, the conversation around sex has evolved, and many in our 50 plus age group are more willing to push boundaries and try things they never would have considered before. Whether it's exploring tantra, as popularized by figures like Sting, or simply being open to longer lasting and more varied sexual encounters, there's a greater propensity for experimentation. While these topics might be controversial or even sensational to some, they are paramount discussions for those looking to break away from the norms of their past and embrace a more liberated and fulfilling sex life. Addressing these desires and curiosities head-on can make for a more engaging and relevant conversation in today's realm of dating and relationships.

Achieving Exclusivity

#126 Scheduling Sex: To Plan Or Not To Plan?

Exploring the Idea: Scheduling Intimacy in Relationships

One interesting aspect of relationships to explore is the concept of scheduling sex. I personally don't adhere to a strict timetable, still, it's a topic that generates diverse opinions. I do believe that spontaneity and desire are indispensable ingredients for a fulfilling sex life, however, for some couples, particularly those with busy schedules or changing libido due to age, planning intimacy might be a viable option. If you are struggling to find the time or prioritize intimacy, adding it to the calendar may be a workable solution to at least trial.

Finding Balance: What's Considered "Healthy" in Intimacy?

What is most important is striking a balance that works for both partners. People will often ask me how frequent is "healthy" for a relationship and while there is no right or wrong, a universal guideline of two to three times a week for sex or some form of physical intimacy is a good barometer. With that, keep in mind that what constitutes "intimacy" can evolve over time and vary greatly between individuals.

Ultimately, open communication and mutual respect are key to maintaining a satisfying sexual relationship at any age. Voice what you want. And if your significant other isn't speaking up—ask.

#127 What Men Need To Make It Work

Adults undoubtedly bring unique perspectives to relationships. Over the years of guiding individuals towards love, I've identified key factors that contribute to fulfilling partnerships for men.

Support and Encouragement

Men thrive on feeling valued and appreciated. Whether it's a new career venture or a personal goal, offering support and encouragement can significantly boost their confidence. Celebrate their achievements and be their biggest cheerleader.

Acceptance and Respect

Every man is unique, and it's important to accept him for who he is. Avoid trying to mold him into your ideal partner. Respect his individuality, interests, and opinions.

Achieving Exclusivity

Effective Communication

Listening actively and expressing your feelings openly are vital components of a healthy relationship. Encourage him to do the same. Effective communication involves both speaking and understanding.

Physical and Emotional Intimacy

While physical intimacy is fundamental to a relationship's success, emotional connection is equally important. This includes acts of service, quality time, words of affirmation, and physical touch.

Shared Values and Goal

A sturdy foundation is built on shared values and life aspirations. Individual differences are healthy, however, aligning on core principles can lead to a more fulfilling partnership.

By understanding and addressing these fundamental needs, women can create a stronger, more fulfilling connection with their male partners. Every relationship is unique, and honest and unfettered communication is key to navigating its complexities.

#128 What Women Need to Make It Work

Conversely, here are 10 things I hear regularly from women about what they want in men:

Confidence

A man who's comfortable in his own skin is incredibly attractive. Women are drawn to men who exude self-confidence without being arrogant or vain. This involves understanding your worth, believing in your abilities, and not needing external validation. It also includes accepting rejection or criticism with composure and not letting it affect your self-esteem.

Self-care

Self-care is vital at every stage of life, but it becomes even more important as we age. We desire a man who prioritizes his health and overall well-being, including both physical and mental aspects. This includes maintaining a balanced diet, getting regular physical activity, and managing stress. It goes without saying that it involves good personal appearance, grooming, and hygiene.

Achieving Exclusivity

Don't neglect these aspects just because you're in a relationship. And, by the way, we don't want to hear about your aches and pains or upcoming knee replacement on the first few dates (or maybe ever). Okay, if you're madly in love, of course we'll bring you goodies during the knee replacement!

Reliability

Reliability is not boring. Our children need it, and so do our friends. Flakiness and inconsistency are major turn-offs! We're looking for a guy who's reliable, honest, and keeps his word. That means arriving when you say you will, honoring your promises, and being present when she needs a shoulder to lean on. Consistency is key—no mixed signals or ghosting for days!

Chrissy's Story

Chrissy was in a two-year relationship (previously married for 15 years and widowed young). The first year with Thomas was fantastic, with the only thing that made her nervous being some one- to two-week breaks in conversations, texts, and seeing each other. He was working intensely and "stressed," as he'd say when he jumped back into the picture. This started to irritate her as she had the summer free, and they'd made weekend travel plans he had to cancel at the last minute. It happens to all of us, right? But four trips in a row?

Andrea McGinty

The problem: Sometimes we lose our objectivity in a relationship. Her friends warned her—why wasn't he doing what he said he'd do? Then, she found she was making 100% of the plans. Summer of year two was the end. They had planned a seven-day vacation to Capri and Naples together—two days before...well, you know the story. Surprise, surprise, when she came to me, number one on her list of needs was someone who did what they said they would do, when they said they would! Chrissy didn't settle, and she's been in a happy relationship with Michael for the past seven months. Never settle for less.

Never Compare Us to a Younger Woman

The majority of my male clients (around 85%) prefer dating a woman within five years of their age and are respectful and don't do this. Thankfully, most men prefer the love of a mature woman who knows how to handle her man. He recognizes that women of a similar age are the women he can relate to since they share a common demographic.

If a man ever says to you after the third or fourth date, "Do you ever do intermittent fasting? I do and I dropped 15 pounds—you might want to try it." What? This happened to Maura, a 48-year-old client who smartly exited the dinner party they were at and called an Uber.

Achieving Exclusivity

Ah, Carrie, a lovely 63-year-old client of mine, was asked by a man on a first date if she wore a bikini, what type, and if she ever went topless at the beach. He said his last girlfriend had a great "rack" and often did. She quickly said goodbye to him, and she's been dating a 58-year-old man for the past eight months.

No Game Playing

Let's get straight to the point: no more games, please! We've reached that fabulous age where we're just too savvy and a bit too tired for the dating circus. Our time is valuable, and we'd much rather invest it in finding someone truly special than in playing around.

Emotional Intelligence

It's all about juggling your own feelings while tuning into others. Remember, these are broad tendencies, and individual preferences vary. Effective communication and mutual understanding are key to building a lasting and fulfilling relationship with a woman.

Andrea McGinty

#129 Looking At Labels

**Introducing Your Partner:
Navigating Labels with Ease**

So, you're in a relationship—maybe it's just starting, or maybe it's quite serious! Labels often come up, not within the relationship itself, but when you introduce your partner to others: friends, family, colleagues, children, acquaintances, etc.
What are the best words to use? It's 100% about what makes both of you feel comfortable.
Personally, in my 20s, the terms "boyfriend" and later "fiancé" were fine and common (1990s). I think back to when my now husband Jeff, two months into our dating/relationship—geez I didn't even know what to call it at that point! Anyways, he introduced me to his basketball crew at the Miami Arena: "This is Andrea"—no label. Since he had never introduced any woman to them before (lucky me?), they understood right away that I must be serious.
Later, when Jeff and I became a "thing" in our late 50s and early 60s, "boyfriend" and "girlfriend" felt... juvenile. "Partner" seemed too cold, like a business partner, or a term more commonly used in same-sex relationships. "Significant other"? It's just a mouthful.

Achieving Exclusivity

On the other hand, my ex-husband Daniel has been in a relationship for the past three years, and they live together. While he has no plans to marry again, Daniel and Deborah refer to each other as "husband" and "wife" when introducing themselves.

What's Right for You?

Ultimately, it's about what feels right to you. I didn't feel the need for a label. When talking to my family and close girlfriends about Jeff, I'd say, "Guess what, I have a boyfriend," and we'd all smile. I had to describe him somehow, so they'd know he wasn't just a "friend."

Jeff, on the other hand, is more reserved—he's from Boston, after all. When he first took me to the Cape (Cape Cod) to meet his family, he told them he was bringing a "friend." His children found this hilarious, and soon his dad started referring to me as "Jeff's friend."

You set the stage—you decide the label, or maybe you don't use one at all. A couple holding hands, with the man saying, "This is Susan," makes it pretty clear that it's not a work colleague or a non-romantic situation.

Common Labels

1. Other half

2. Sweetheart or beau (used in a playful way)

3. Girlfriend/boyfriend

4. Partner

5. Significant other (How do you say this with a straight face and not giggle? I couldn't!)

6. Fiancé

7. "This is Michael—we just got engaged" (Well, that says it all!)

8. "This is my date, Thomas."

Achieving Exclusivity

So, when do you apply a label? It can be an uncomfortable discussion, and many couples never have this chat. One might say "boyfriend," while the other says "friend" or "partner."

For those over 45+, around the three-month mark might be a good time to have a quick, fun chat about it, if needed. By then, you're probably seeing each other 2-3 times a week and are exclusive.

Why do we need labels? Are they just a societal nicety or rooted in insecurity? I'd simply go with, "I'd like you to meet Ryan," or "This is my date, Ryan."

#130 Tests, Quizzes, and Insights On Love Languages

**Love Languages:
What They Mean and Why They Matter**

You may often come across statements like, "My LL is quality time," and wonder, "What does that even mean?" Yes, these are commonly mentioned on dating sites and apps, or from others when a relationship gets rolling. The most popular is the Love Languages quiz. You can take a free test here—it's fun! But more importantly, if you take it honestly, you might learn something valuable about yourself, and you'll definitely understand what others are talking about online.

Andrea McGinty

A love language is a specific way individuals express and receive love. The concept, introduced by Dr. Gary Chapman, identifies five primary love languages: words of affirmation, acts of service, receiving gifts, quality time, and physical touch. Each person has one or more preferred love languages that make them feel most loved and appreciated.

Understanding and speaking your partner's love language enhances communication, strengthens emotional connections, and fosters a deeper, more fulfilling relationship by ensuring both partners feel valued and understood. *(This paragraph is adapted from another source and could use your own voice.)*

Are there other personality tests out there? Of course. Myers-Briggs, for example, when someone says, "I'm an INTJ." Is it as common? Not really—it's more popular in the business world. StrengthsFinder, developed by Gallup, is super interesting, but also less commonly used online. Of these "Big 3," StrengthsFinder is my personal favorite, but it's a bit of a commitment since you need to buy the book, read it, and use the code for a deep analysis of yourself and your compatibility with others.

But Love Languages? That's just fun!

Achieving Exclusivity

Why Stick to Love Languages?

Let's stick with the most popular: Love Languages. To give you an example, here's Caroline, a 57-year-old client of mine in Washington, DC, who kindly shared her experience:

>1. Her initial Love Languages quiz as a single, taken just before she became my client.

>2. Her quiz results after six months of being serious with Michael.

>3. Michael's Love Languages quiz, taken at the six-month mark in their relationship.

They are now happily married as of April 2024. Did this quiz predict their love and marriage? No! But did they learn about each other? Absolutely.

Here Are the Results

1. Caroline (Single, before Michael): *Primary Love Language: Receiving Gifts* Caroline finds deep connection through receiving gifts. Tokens of affection are a tangible expression of love for her. She cherishes the time and effort someone puts into selecting and presenting a gift, remembering even small tokens for years due to the emotional attachment.

2. Caroline (after 6 months with Michael): *Primary Love Language: Acts of Service* Thoughtful, selfless actions quickly win Caroline's heart. When a loved one goes out of their way to make her life easier, she feels deeply connected. For her, actions speak louder than words, and acts of service fill her "love tank."

3. Michael's Love Languages quiz (after 6 months with Caroline). *Primary Love Language: Quality Tim.* Michael values undivided attention and meaningful time spent together. Whether through deep conversations or shared experiences, quality time makes him feel deeply loved and prioritized.

So, we have Quality Time and Acts of Service—different, but complementary. Did this guarantee their relationship's success? Of course not. But it helped them learn more about each other. Now, take a look back at Caroline's first quiz—it was all about gifts, right?

Are we going to marry someone based on quiz results? No. But we're never too old to learn more about ourselves!

Should you include your love language results on your online dating profile? That's up to you. Personally, I didn't, and I don't advise my clients to either. But if you see someone who has, and you've taken the quiz, feel free to share your results if you think it will spark interest!

#131 Building Trust, Communication, and a Shared Future

It takes work—don't take these tenants for granted.

Navigating Trust After Heartbreak

Tim's 28-year marriage ended after his wife cheated, and after three years of being divorced (and a bit of therapy), he came to me as a client. Was trust still an issue? Absolutely. But we tackled it head-on during our coaching calls, especially when he hit the 4-month mark with a woman he really liked—Mila.

Now, Tim's the analytical, quiet type. We could have gone round and round, analyzing every detail for weeks. But I knew what he really needed was to open up to Mila and be honest about his fears. The result? He took the leap, had the talk with Mila, and they worked through it together. Now, everything's coming up roses for Tim!

Envisioning a Shared Future

Trust and open communication are the bedrock of any successful relationship. Sharing thoughts, feelings, and desires honestly creates a safe space for both partners to express themselves without fear of judgment. Building trust involves reliability, consistency, and keeping promises. It's about creating a foundation of security and confidence in the relationship.

Beyond the present, envisioning a shared future together is critical. Whether it's discussing life goals, career aspirations, or family planning, couples who align their long-term visions tend to have stronger bonds. This doesn't mean rigid adherence to a predetermined plan, but rather a shared direction that allows for flexibility and growth.

Achieving Exclusivity

#132 Clean Up the Camera Roll and Old Chats

**Trust and Communication:
The Bedrock of Strong Relationships**

When you're getting serious with someone, eliminate any unnecessary baggage that could create tension or awkwardness. This means cleaning up your phone—deleting old chats, photos, or anything else that might upset your partner. Even if something on your phone is harmless, the fact that it's still there can lead to unnecessary drama. For instance, if your partner sees a random notification from someone they don't know, it could spark doubt or insecurity, even if there's no reason for it.

I've seen this happen before. I once had a female client in Los Angeles who was in a newly exclusive relationship. Both were in their early forties and traveled a lot for work but were very much committed to their future together. Late one Saturday night, they were lying in bed watching a movie on his iPad, and a Facebook Messenger notification popped up from a girl he had obviously been talking to.

Andrea McGinty

A few minutes later, she started Facebook calling. Flustered, he quickly muted the call. Neither said a word about it. They continued watching the movie. My client figured it was probably remnants of old flirty texts that he hadn't properly shut down since going exclusive. However, she was clearly uncomfortable about what had happened but swept it under the rug. The relationship didn't last.

On another occasion, a friend Ebony and her partner Rick, who were together about three years at this point and had a baby, were saying their good nights in bed when he opened his phone to check the weather for the following day. As Rick unlocked his phone, a bunch of widgets showed up on the phone—including a bathroom selfie of another woman that Ebony saw for a split second before he dismissed it, too quick to determine if she was topless. (But the inkling was that she was...) Rick said nothing and went to sleep, and Ebony lay awake wondering what to do, processing what she had just seen.

Achieving Exclusivity

The following morning, she asked what the photo was about—unable to hide her distress. Rick calmly acknowledged the photograph and explained earnestly that he had 35,000 photos on his phone dating back 14 years that he had never cleaned up or deleted. He reiterated that the photo was taken many years before they got together and that it came up as a camera roll memory—which can certainly happen. Ebony had no reason to doubt or suspect her partner of any wandering, but the photo had really thrown her for a loop. The couple resolved the situation, but it created unnecessary upset and distrust in the meantime.

The Power of Open Communication

The lesson? Please clean up the tech and social media before it's a problem. Such situations can be easily avoided by taking some proactive steps when you're entering an exclusive relationship (obviously on the basis that you have nothing to hide!):

1. Clear Out Old Chats and Photos. Go through your messages and delete anything that might be misconstrued. This doesn't mean hiding things but removing unnecessary clutter that could cause misunderstandings.

2. Turn Off Notifications. Turn off notifications that might pop up unexpectedly, especially when you're spending time with your partner. It's a straightforward way to avoid creating an awkward moment.

3. Organize Your Social Media . Review your social media accounts, clean up your DMs, and consider unfollowing or muting accounts that could make your partner uncomfortable.

4. Be Transparent. If something does come up, address it immediately. Don't let minor issues fester. If your partner sees something on your phone that makes them uncomfortable, have an open conversation about it right then and there.

Set Boundaries . Agree on boundaries together. Maybe it's about not texting others late at night or being mindful of who you interact with on social media.

By taking these steps, you can avoid unnecessary drama and build a stronger foundation of trust in your relationship. It's not about hiding things; it's about being respectful and considerate as you move into a more serious relationship stage.

#133 Dealing with Social Media Use Dating and in A Relationship

Most people have some social media presence, and in the 45 plus age group, it tends to be Facebook and Instagram. Here are a few frequently asked questions:

Achieving Exclusivity

Frequently Asked Questions

1. Should I link my social media to a dating app? No, you should not. There is enough information on your dating app or site, and there's no need to get so personal so fast. If someone asks for your social media before meeting you, say no. If they insist, block or delete them.

2. When should I change my relationship status online? Many social media platforms offer status options like Single, Divorced, Widowed, In a Relationship, Engaged, etc. Most people, even in an exclusive relationship, don't make changes to their status. However, if you'd like to post a wedding or engagement photo, it's appropriate to change your status to Married or Engaged.

3. Can I post photos of my new relationship online? Not without their permission. Some people don't use social media for various reasons. For instance, I have a high-profile athlete client who is currently dating someone. At a party where a few photos were taken, he asked her not to post them—not because he didn't like her (they're still dating), but because it's not his thing. He has a PR firm that handles such matters, and as he mentioned, it was much too early in the relationship for that.

Another client of mine, a woman from a small town, was asked by her boyfriend if it was okay to post photos of them paddleboarding. She said no, even though she's on social media, because her children (early teens) don't yet know about the relationship. Makes sense, right? Plus, it's the polite thing to do! While many people are fine with posting photos, always ask first and be respectful.

4. You break up–should you delete photos?
Here are a few considerations:

- If it's someone you've been dating for the past year or two, it's a personal choice. You probably don't need to delete photos unless it was a horrible breakup. However, if you changed your status to "In a Relationship," change it back to your previous status.

- As for your past, we all have one! Maybe you were married for 20 years, and there are photos of you, your ex, and the kids—should you delete them? No. This is part of your history, part of your life. Okay, your marriage didn't last forever—that's okay. There were still happy memories. For fun, while writing this book, I went back and saw I've been a Facebook member since 2008. Yes, of course, my ex-husband is in some photos, along with the kids. Would I delete these happy memories of Disney, beach vacations, and laying in a crypt in Egypt? No way!

Achieving Exclusivity

Do's and Don'ts with Social Media and Dating

1. Don't add them as a friend or follow them before a date—or even after 3-4 dates (you'll look like a stalker).

2. Don't like any of their photos before a first date—it's creepy.

3. It's okay to check if you have any common friends.

4. Take what you see online with a grain of salt—are we all happy 24/7?

5. Don't overshare online (it's a turn-off).

Andrea McGinty

#134 Talk Money

Want to Talk about Dating, Money, and Your Relationship? Most Don't...

Yes, you *must* talk about money.

I'm not suggesting you do this on the first date—or even the second. But it absolutely needs to be discussed once you're in the "serious relationship" or "heading towards long-term commitment" phase. I know it's a tad awkward, but it is a non-negotiable for a mature, lasting relationship. (Interestingly, more people feel comfortable talking about religion or politics than discussing personal finances.) Still, don't linger too long avoiding the topic or assume you already know the answers. You need to be sure because here's the bottom line: it's the third leading cause of breakups, after "incompatibility" and "infidelity."

Yes, financial issues can be a significant source of stress in relationships. According to the American Institute of CPAs, 73% of married or cohabiting Americans experience relationship tension due to money decisions. Financial tensions can escalate quickly—who needs these kinds of problems at this stage in life?

Achieving Exclusivity

As we accumulate more wealth, this conversation becomes increasingly crucial. Think back to when you were in your 20s or early 30s, just getting married—talking about your wealth (or lack thereof) was simpler. Didn't we all seem to know how much our friends made back then? We were all starting out.

When I first got married at 30 (we were married for 24 years), I was hanging on by a financial thread. I'd just started a company (*It's Just Lunch*), and every penny I earned went back into growing the business. The man I married was a partner at a law firm, earning an impressive salary for a 32-year-old. We had an open conversation about money. It was straightforward: I had none; he had some. We agreed to keep separate checking and savings accounts (mine had zero savings, of course), along with a joint account where we each contributed a set amount each month. We also agreed that any purchase of over $1,000 for shared living spaces, like art or furniture, had to be mutually approved.

When you're younger, financial decisions are simpler. The 20s through 40s are often focused on acquiring things—homes, nicer cars, maybe even a second home or a boat. You're climbing the financial ladder. More assets equal more at stake.

Andrea McGinty

But let's fast forward to the 2020s. Having more wealth is definitely a plus in the dating market. Yet, the very thing that can make someone attractive to many people can also end a relationship. Many people lack the communication skills needed to handle financial disagreements in a relationship. Or they might communicate well about everything *except* money, which still wrenches open a fatal gap in the bond.

So, what should you do? Go full transparency on finances? Share the last seven years of tax returns? Conduct an IRS-style audit?

No, there are easier ways to navigate this all-important conversation.

Here Are My Tips

> **1. Timing matters**. The key times to have financial talks are before moving in together, when starting a committed relationship, and definitely before marriage. This isn't a discussion for the first month of dating—though by then, you'll likely start to notice your partner's spending habits. People tend to be on their best behavior during the first month or two of dating, so it may not be an accurate picture.

Achieving Exclusivity

2. Don't spring it on them. This isn't a casual "By the way, let's talk about money" conversation. It's an important discussion that too many people delay until the last minute. Again, don't wait. Kindly let your partner know you'd like to sit down for an hour or two to discuss that dreaded topic—money. This isn't the time to talk about where to live or plan your dream vacation, but rather how you both intend to manage finances as a couple. Do you need to show financial statements? Probably not.

For example, one of my clients, Mike, 58, a successful business executive who travels extensively, accumulated a lot of airline miles and hotel points. Before marrying Lana, a retired creative director who now focuses on painting, she brought up how to handle day-to-day expenses, given that her income is currently minimal, although she has other assets. The outcome? They decided to live in Lana's mortgage-free home, split monthly expenses like HOA fees and utilities, and for their big trips (this year's destinations are Sri Lanka and Norway), Mike covers the flights and hotels using his points.

3. Be honest. If you have debt or ongoing alimony payments, share this with your partner. You might be head over heels in love and ready to commit, but transparency matters big-time. Don't hide things. That includes being honest about what you do own—shadiness never bodes well.

Take Lizette, 51, a sales executive who loves to shop. From shoes at Bergdorf's to Etsy and Amazon finds, her home is delivery central—every day. Her partner Chris, 56, a CPA, has zero interest in shopping. Early in their relationship, Lizette set up a UPS Store box to receive her packages so she could sneak them into their home at night when Chris wasn't around. Of course, he eventually found out. Chris couldn't have cared less about what she bought, but he was upset that she felt the need to hide it from him. For Chris, it was about trust and transparency, not the spending itself. They worked it out, and now Liz gets her packages delivered to their home—no more wondering what else she might be hiding.

Achieving Exclusivity

4. Plan for the future. As we age, certain realities become unavoidable. If you intend to leave your estate to children, others, or your new spouse, handle this responsibly. Before moving in together or getting married, ensure these documents are in place:

- A notarized will

- A prenuptial or postnuptial agreement if significant assets are involved (consult an attorney or estate planner)

- Trusts, life insurance, living wills, and directives You want to make things easy for your children or partner, leaving no questions unanswered.

This is a personal business I'm in—helping people navigate their love lives! So perhaps I tend to overshare, but this is me: My dad passed away recently, and he was incredibly organized (in addition to being an amazing man). Each of his six children received an annual email for the last five years, detailing where his assets were, amounts, etc., making it easy for my brother to handle the estate. And in each letter, he also expressed how much he loved us.

In other words, don't underestimate the importance of discussing finances in your dating life. Engaging in money conversations—early and often—can actually strengthen your relationship. Research shows that couples who openly discuss their financial situations tend to report higher levels of happiness compared to those who avoid the topic. Who wouldn't want to start a relationship on a positive note?

Suggested Questions to Help Start the Discussion

Not every question will apply to every couple, so choose the ones that work for you:

1. Are you more of a spender or a saver?

2. Do you keep a monthly budget?

3. What is your annual income?

4. How much do you typically spend each month?

5. How do you usually spend your disposable income?

6. What's the most money you've ever spent at one time?

Achieving Exclusivity

7. Do you think it's important to ask for my permission before making a large purchase?

8. Which expenses would you cut to reduce overall spending?

9. Should we split utilities and other expenses equally, or according to our incomes?

10. Should we open a joint bank account or keep our finances separate?

11. What would you do if you received lottery winnings, an inheritance, or another unexpected windfall?

Debt and Credit Questions

In a relationship, each partner's debt and credit score can impact their shared financial future. To better understand how your partner handles credit, consider these questions:

1. What are your credit scores?

2. How many credit cards do you have?

3. Do you know the outstanding balance of each card?

4. How much debt do you currently have?

5. Do you owe money to friends or family?

6. Have you ever filed for bankruptcy?

Achieving Exclusivity

Children and Family Questions

Family-related financial topics can be tricky but are particularly crucial if you plan to maintain a healthy long-term relationship.

1. Do you owe alimony or child support to a previous partner?

2. Do you plan to pursue further education for yourself now or in the future?

3. Would you lend money to a friend or relative in need?

4. Do you plan to support your parents or other relatives as they age?

5. Did your parents teach you any important lessons about money?

Retirement and Investing Questions

If you and your partner hope to spend your golden years together, you need to agree on your expectations leading up to and during retirement.

1. How do you envision your retirement?

2. Where do you hope to retire?

3. What's your ideal retirement age?

Andrea McGinty

#135 More Tips for Lasting Relationships

We've all experienced that electric spark—that instant attraction we hope will endure. Or perhaps it was a slow burn that eventually ignited a passionate relationship. While I typically focus on dating (given that over 60% of my clients are single), I want to share some insights on maintaining a thriving relationship. These tips can also be beneficial for those still navigating the dating scene.

Love at First Sight is a Rom-Com Myth

The notion of finding love unexpectedly is a common misconception. It can happen, but relying on serendipity is a risky strategy. Building a lasting relationship requires effort and intention. Instead of passively waiting, actively participate in creating opportunities to connect with potential partners.

Achieving Exclusivity

Seek Shared Interests

Joining groups or activities aligned with your passions is a fantastic way to meet like-minded people. My client Trina, for instance, discovered a vibrant community of artists when she joined a glassblowing workshop. This newfound sense of belonging contributed to her overall happiness and ultimately led to a meaningful relationship.

Cultivate Positivity

Happy people tend to attract others. A positive outlook can be contagious and make you more appealing to potential partners. If you're struggling with negative patterns, consider seeking professional help to overcome obstacles.

Balance Similarities and Differences

Shared values and compatibility are important, yet differences can also add excitement and depth to a relationship. Prioritize communication, common values, and chemistry. A solid foundation in these areas can help navigate potential challenges.

Prioritize Self-Care

Maintaining your own identity and interests is vital for a healthy relationship. Spending time with friends, family, and pursuing personal hobbies enriches your life and prevents feelings of dependency.

Whether you're happily coupled up or looking to find that special someone, remember that building and maintaining a fulfilling relationship takes effort and self-awareness.

BLUE
embodies
trust and stability,
key qualities when
Navigating Family Dynamics with new relationships in which you're aiming for harmony and connection.

chapter 11
Navigating Family Dynamics

#136 Introducing a New Partner To Your Children

**Timing is Everything:
When to Introduce Your Partner
to Your Children**

Introducing a new partner to your children is a delicate matter, influenced heavily by the children's ages and the dynamics of the parents' relationship. Consider the age gap between yourself and your partner, as well as the age of your children. A significant age difference can be jarring for teenagers. Distinguish between casual dating and a committed relationship before involving children. Introducing them to someone you've only dated a few times is inappropriate.

Navigating Family Dynamics

**Personal Insight:
The First Meeting**

Timing is crucial. Allow your relationship to mature before introducing your children. I would definitely advise waiting until the relationship is defined as exclusive by both parties. Two to three months can be a reasonable timeframe to assess compatibility and commitment. Children are perceptive and may pick up on underlying tensions or uncertainties. Their emotional well-being should always be a priority.

I'll never forget meeting Jeff's kids for the first time. We had been trying to coordinate a dinner at the Beach Club, but it always seemed like someone had a scheduling conflict.

One day, I stopped by Jeff's house and met his 19-year-old son and 22-year-old daughter. It was a casual introduction, and my dog Luna helped break the ice with Jeff's dog, Lily.

Andrea McGinty

#137 Balancing Dating and Family Responsibilities

Navigating Family Life and Dating in Your 50s and 60s

Juggling dating and family life can be complex, especially in your 50s and 60s. If you have younger children, the challenges are magnified. Important family events like graduations or weddings can complicate new relationships. Deciding whether to include a new partner in these events depends on the relationship's stage and the potential impact on everyone involved.

Teenagers are usually less concerned about their parents' dating lives, but introducing multiple partners too soon can create confusion and instability for children. Prioritize your children's emotional well-being and avoid introducing them to casual dating partners.

Balancing Personal Happiness and Family Obligations

Finding the right balance between your personal life and family responsibilities is essential. Of course, it is important to consider your children's feelings. However, it's equally essential to prioritize your own happiness and well-being. Your children will eventually grow up and become independent, while your romantic partner could be a lifelong companion.

Each situation is unique. Open communication with your children and careful consideration of everyone's feelings are critical considerations when navigating this delicate balance.

#138 Build A Supportive Family Environment

Family in Your Later Years

Creating a supportive family environment in your later years involves cultivating a sense of belonging, respect, and shared experiences. This can be achieved by:

1. Open Communication: Fostering open and honest dialogue with your partner and family members is vital. Sharing thoughts, feelings, and expectations creates a foundation of trust and understanding.

2. Shared Values and Goals: Aligning shared values and life goals strengthens the bond between partners and their respective families. This creates a sense of purpose and direction for the family unit.

3. Quality Time: Prioritizing quality time together, whether through shared activities, holidays, or simply spending quiet moments, deepens connections and strengthens relationships.

4. Respect for Individuality: While building a shared life, it's important to respect each individual's needs, interests, and independence. This fosters a sense of autonomy and appreciation within the family.

5. Creating New Traditions: Establishing new family traditions can help create a sense of unity and belonging. These traditions can be as simple as regular family dinners or as elaborate as annual vacations.

6. Supporting Each Other: Offering emotional support, encouragement, and practical assistance to family members demonstrates care and strengthens the family bond.

By focusing on these elements, you can build a supportive and fulfilling family environment that brings joy and satisfaction to everyone involved.

INDIGO suggests introspection and intuition, guiding you through **Special Consideerations When Dating** whether health-related, personal history, or other.

chapter 12
Special Considerations When Dating

#136 Introducing a New Partner To Your Children

This topic has come up several times with my clients. For instance, I had a female client, Tara, age 56, from Louisville, Kentucky, who was recently widowed. She had spent the last 10 years caring for her husband, who had muscular dystrophy. Their 28-year-old son also has the same condition and lives at home with her.

How Should This Be Handled in Dating?

Tara wanted to include information about her husband's and son's illnesses in her dating profile, so potential partners would know upfront, and she could weed out those who might be freaked out by her situation. However, I disagreed. Sensitive topics like these shouldn't be shared on dating sites from the outset.

Special Considerations When Dating

Here's My Approach

1. Profile Content: Write a profile that *does not* include this information. This isn't about being dishonest but rather about protecting your privacy and allowing the relationship to develop naturally.

2. First Date Conversation: It's natural to mention being widowed on a first date but keep it brief. You could say something like, "My husband passed away after a long illness, and I'm excited to start dating again." Avoid going into details or specifics—you're still getting to know the person.

3. Discussing Special Needs: After about three dates, if you feel there's potential for an ongoing relationship, you can begin to share more personal details. For example, you might explain that your son attends a special education facility five days a week for eight hours.

4. Establishing Boundaries: Until you really know someone, it's unfair to bring them into your personal situations right away. They need to get to know *you* first.

5. Self-Discovery: After years of caregiving, this might be a time for you to rediscover yourself. Your initial goal in dating could simply be to explore what's out there and enjoy getting your feet wet in the dating world again.

Andrea McGinty

#140 Dating As A Widow or Widower

Navigating the dating sector after the loss of a spouse is both a brave and tender quest. Whether your partner passed away recently or several years ago, deciding to seek companionship again can bring up a mix of emotions—ranging from excitement to guilt, or even apprehension. Everyone's timeline and readiness are unique. While the way forward might feel uncertain, it can also lead to a renewed sense of joy and fulfillment.

I've had the privilege of working with many widows and widowers. What I've found is that those who had happy, loving relationships are often the most optimistic about finding love again. They know what a good partnership looks like and believe it's possible to experience that kind of connection once more. Here are a few things to keep in mind:

1. Positive Outlook. Widows and widowers are often my favorite clients. Over 30 years of doing this, I've found they generally had happy relationships, which gives them a positive outlook on love and companionship. They know what a good relationship feels like, and they expect it again—an attitude that's wonderful to work with.

Special Considerations When Dating

2. Timing is Personal. No one can dictate when Just a few weeks later, he married a 70-year-old woman who had never been married. It was a heartwarming story that reminds us there's no right or wrong time to find love.

3. Avoid Constant Comparisons. Talking about how amazing your late spouse was can signal that you're not ready to date. If this is the case, it's okay to take more time to grieve.

4. Think About the Future. Consider what you want in your next season of life and what kind of partner would fit into that vision.

5. Telling Your Children. Wait until you're truly serious about someone before introducing them to your children. Occasionally, children may struggle with the idea of a new relationship due to unresolved grief or concerns about inheritance. However, it's important for them to understand that their parents have many years left to live, and companionship can greatly enhance their quality of life. You do deserve to prioritize you.

Andrea McGinty

A Story of Renewed Love: Finding Companionship After Loss

As I mentioned in the introduction, my dad has a beautiful story of finding love again. My father, Jack, was a man of deep faith and unwavering routines and faced the most profound loss when my mother passed away. For six long years, he navigated life without her, finding solace in his daily rituals and the familiar echoes of our family home. But as time flowed on, so too did the possibility of new beginnings.

It was during a high school reunion that fate intervened. There stood Ginnie, his high school sweetheart— her uplifting smile conjuring images of innocence and youthful dreams. Ginnie had entered the convent right after high school, dedicating two decades to a life of service. It was a life filled with prayer and silence, but also one marked by unfulfilled longing. After leaving the convent, she married a man who already had five children, stepping into the role of a stepmother.

In many ways, Jack and Ginnie's reunion felt like something out of a storybook, reminiscent of *The Sound of Music*, where a nun discovers love after a life of devotion. As my father's children, we welcomed this unexpected turn with open hearts, thrilled to see him smiling again. Ginnie lived in Victoria, Canada—so it was a bit of a hike from my father's base in Cleveland, Ohio. Nevertheless, the regular trips to and from became a bridge for their love, with visits spanning months as they nurtured their rekindled romance until dad eventually felt comfortable enough to relocate.

But before Ginnie entered his life, I noticed that my father had begun to explore the notion of love anew with much more of an open mind than even I could have imagined. He frequented the gym, and one day, as he wiped sweat from his brow, he called me with excitement.

"You won't believe it! There's this really cute Jewish woman I keep seeing on the treadmill," he exclaimed. "We talk about so much! She's just so adorable."

**Embracing New Chapters:
Love Without Boundaries**

I couldn't help but smile at his newfound openness, a reminder that love knows no boundaries and transcends the stereotypes we often cling to. It was this attitude that, I believe, led him back to Ginnie. I often think of how happy they were together—and I am so grateful he spent the twilight of his life with a partner he loved—which makes me all the more saddened when clients tell me how their children do not support them on the dating scene. Do these kids really want to look after their folks forever? Do they never want to see them smile again?

Still, I reiterate—this is a personal decision. When you are ready, put the naysayers aside, and do what feels right to you. I hold onto the hope that no matter the obstacles, companionship is a beautiful adventure worth pursuing.

#141 Dealing with Past Divorces and Emotional Baggage

When it comes to dating after divorce, the conversation often centers around "emotional baggage." But let's shift that perspective—what if we called it what it really is: life experience? Each of us carries a wealth of knowledge from our past, and that experience can make us wiser, smarter, and more attuned to the alarm bells that may have eluded us in our younger years.

Shifting the Perspective: Life Experience Over Emotional Baggage

Those who have amicably navigated a divorce tend to re-enter the dating world sooner and with a more positive outlook. They've closed one period of their lives, ready to embrace the next with open hearts. On the other hand, if you've faced a contentious divorce that dragged on, take the time to process those emotions—whether through personal reflection, a divorce support group, or one-on-one therapy.

Reflecting on my own relationship sojourn, after 24 years of marriage, my divorce was relatively pleasant—but it was still a significant transition. I chose to attend a church support group focused on divorce, where we met weekly to share our experiences and work through a guided workbook. What struck me most was the gratitude I felt after hearing others' stories; mine wasn't as tumultuous as some. That single meeting left me feeling surprisingly light, even though I had contemplated this decision for five years before finally making it.

**Navigating Divorce:
A Path to Positivity or Processing**

Here are some tips for those venturing back into the dating sphere:

1. Acknowledge Your Rustiness: You might feel out of practice, and that's okay! Recognizing it is the first step to overcoming it.

2. Engage in Activities You Love: Start by meeting new people through hobbies or interests that genuinely excite you. This not only fosters conversation but also encourages personal growth.

Special Considerations When Dating

3. Give Yourself Time: After a year, many divorcees feel ready to date again. The landscape of dating has evolved significantly since your 20s.

4. Consider Professional Guidance: With the plethora of dating sites and apps—over 1,400 of them—hiring a professional can help you navigate the options without feeling overwhelmed.

5. Avoid Speaking Negatively About Your Ex: If asked why your marriage ended, a simple, "I prefer not to discuss that on the first date. Have you seen the latest movie?" can redirect the conversation without dwelling on the past.

6. Discuss Your Children: It's perfectly fine to mention your kids and their ages but avoid diving into specific challenges or issues, especially if they're sensitive.

7. Set Boundaries on Personal Topics: Your date likely isn't interested in hearing about your problems.

8. Trust Yourself Over Others: Friends and family may have opinions on whether you're ready to date again, but only you can truly know your readiness.

Let's also rethink the term "emotionally unavailable." Often, this label is thrown around casually, but what it really signifies is a lack of availability for a relationship—not necessarily a reflection of someone's worth or past experiences. In cultures like those of Japan and China, elders are revered for their wisdom and life experiences. It's time we adopt a similar perspective toward ourselves. Rather than seeing our pasts as burdens, we should celebrate the insights and strengths they bring. After all, navigating life's complexities makes us who we are—individuals ready to embrace love once more, with hearts full of understanding and hope.

#142 Finding Love after Major Life Changes

Life is a series of transformations, and each notable change can impact our ability to find love. Many of us are familiar with the emotional toll of death and divorce, other shifts—like job loss, illness, or moving—yet these can still shape our readiness to date.

Here are a few thoughts to ponder.

Special Considerations When Dating

Job Loss:
A Time for Reflection

Losing a job can hit hard, affecting both your self-esteem and finances. Until you regain your footing and find a new role, it's probably best to pause your dating life. Focus on your career and take the time to heal. When one of my clients, Harry, transitioned to the presidency of a major ad agency, we agreed to put his dating membership on hold for a month. He needed that space to acclimate to his new position without the added pressure of dating.

Similarly, I worked with a woman who had just taken over as the director of admissions at an Ivy League school. The learning curve was steep, and the pressures immense. This wasn't the ideal time for her to start dating, as her attention needed to be given to her professional responsibilities.

There are exceptions. If you find yourself in a situation where a job loss frees up your time and isn't a major financial burden, it might present an unexpected opportunity for dating. It's all about your mindset and readiness. If you feel stressed and uncertain about your future, it's best to hit pause and work through those emotions first.

Illness:
Prioritize Your Health

Health challenges, whether recovering from a knee replacement or finishing chemotherapy, are not conducive to dating. No one wants to spend a first date discussing aches and pains or feeling like they need to take care of their date. It's important to wait until you're feeling your best before stepping back into the dating scene. Focus on your recovery and ensure you're in a positive place physically and mentally.

Moving:
A Fresh Start

Moving can be a life-changing event, offering a unique opportunity for romance. Whether relocating across the country or just to a neighboring town, new surroundings bring fresh faces and exciting experiences. You can explore local hotspots and hidden gems simply by going out on dates.

When you move, consider joining dating platforms or engaging in local activities as a way to meet new people. You might feel like you've exhausted your options in your old city, but a new place opens up an entirely different pool of potential partners. The excitement of exploring a new city can reignite your spirit and motivate you to embrace this new chapter of your life.

Special Considerations When Dating

Navigating the dating landscape after major life changes requires self-awareness and consideration. While some changes may signal a time to pause and reflect, others—like moving to a new location—can be the perfect opportunity to dive back into dating. Embrace the journey, focus on your personal growth, and be open to the possibilities that lie ahead. After all, love often blooms when we least expect it, especially during times of transformation.

#143 Adjusting To New Relationship Dynamics

Let's face it: we aren't 20 anymore. The carefree days of partying in bars and clubs have faded, replaced by a different landscape where relationships are often forged in the digital realm. Even though many of us didn't grow up with the internet, we've adapted to its presence in our lives—navigating emails and social media with relative ease. Yet, when it comes to online dating, the transition can feel overwhelming.

Andrea McGinty

Embracing the Modern Dating Landscape: Adjusting to a New Adventure

The biggest change we face today is embracing online dating as an adventure. Many individuals, despite having successful careers and experience with technology, find themselves intimidated by apps like Bumble and Hinge. I've walked numerous clients through this process, and it's often a mix of nerves and uncertainty that holds them back.

To thrive in this unfamiliar environment, cultivate curiosity. The dating landscape is constantly evolving, and you must be willing to learn and adapt. The questions posed on these platforms frequently change, and being flexible can make all the difference. The traditional ways of meeting people—through friends, community events, or serendipitous encounters—are not as prevalent as they once were.

Cultivating Curiosity in the Digital Dating World

View this expedition as an opportunity for growth. Everyone appreciates a person who is still learning, someone who approaches life with an open mind and heart. Welcome the unknown, explore new avenues of connection, and be willing to experiment with different strategies.

Adjusting to these new relationship dynamics may take time, but with a dose of inquisitiveness and a willingness to adapt, you can navigate the online dating world with confidence. After all, love is an adventure waiting to unfold—are you ready to embark on it?

PURPLE represents wisdom and fulfillment, a **Recap on Hope, Love, Fun, and Preparation,** bringing together the lessons you have learned on your journey.

chapter 13
Recap on Hope, Love, Fun—and Preparation
#144 Make That Plan

I know, I know. I mentioned this in the beginning, but I wanted to repeat it once again because it is so important... Love involves a little luck sometimes, I get it. But way more often than not, it comes down to careful and intentional planning and putting your best foot forward with knowledge and grace. Using business principles to approach dating can bring a level of objectivity that can help streamline the process and increase your chances of finding a compatible partner. It may not sound romantic, yet the goal is to find your forever partner, and oftentimes, a strategic approach is what it takes.

Recap on Hope, Love, Fun—and Preparation

Take Tom, for instance, a 60-year-old partner in a law firm who approached dating with an analytical mindset. He treated dating like a sales pipeline, going on three blind dates in the first week, following up with second dates in the second week, and adding new dates to keep the momentum. By the third week, Tom had dates in various stages of development, much like how leads are managed in a sales-driven company.

Sure, Tom's system kept him busy, it wasn't yielding the right results. He had plenty of potential partners, but none truly clicked. That's when I stepped in, helping him refocus on the human aspect of dating rather than just the numbers. The result? Tom is now happily in a relationship with Carina, a 62-year-old ad executive.

This approach can be applied across various aspects of dating. Bottom line?

You Need a Plan

Just like in business, having a clear, strategic plan is a must. The most effective plans in the 2020s are concise, often just a one-pager, which you can easily adapt to your dating goals. This method allows you to balance the structure with spontaneity, ensuring that while you're strategic, you're also open to the natural flow of relationships. Yes, it's important to have a plan, but it's equally crucial to be flexible and take in the sights and sounds of this trek.

And you know what's coming next! Here's a fun exercise: Fill out the below "My Dating Plan." "They" say writing with a pen makes you more committed than tapping away on your mobile. And I give you some real examples too to get you going.

Andrea McGinty

WORKSHEET #12— My Dating Business Plan

#145 Set Goals and Stay The Course

To succeed in dating, you need to approach it with the same mindset that drives successful businesses: goal setting, organization, perseverance, and commitment. Let's draw out our dating notebook.

Elements of Your Dating Notebook

1. Set Clear Goals: Just as Facebook aimed to connect the continents, you need an unclouded vision for your dating journey. Is your goal to date casually, find a long-term relationship (LTR), live together, or get married? Defining your goal will shape your approach and guide your actions. To get started, fill out the Dating Planner/Goal Setter at [insert link here].

Recap on Hope, Love, Fun—and Preparation

2. Stay Organized: Profitable companies thrive on organization, and your dating life should be no different. If your dating profile is chaotic, with dozens of potential matches saved but no clear action plan, it's time to streamline. Make decisive moves by either messaging or deleting these profiles. This not only reduces the clutter but also keeps your focus sharp.

3. Learn from Business Failures: Even the most successful people have faced setbacks. 36 publishers rejected Arianna Huffington's second book. Walt Disney was fired from several jobs, rejected by the army, and went bankrupt before creating his empire. Colonel Sanders failed in various careers before founding KFC. The lesson? Perseverance. They didn't give up after a single failure, and neither should you.

4. Commit to Online Dating: It's surprising how many people give up on online dating (OLD) after just one month. However, those who stay the course, work the system, and maintain a positive attitude often see major rewards. Success in online dating often comes to those who stick with it for at least three months.

Andrea McGinty

As an example, I recently had dinner with four couples, and three out of the four met online through platforms like Match, Bumble, and Our Time. Their online dating adventures ranged from 5 weeks to 2 years, showing that perseverance truly pays off.

The key takeaway? Whether in business or dating, success often comes to those who are clear in their goals, organized in their approach, and relentless in their pursuit.

WORKSHEET #13—
What Are Your Dating Goals?

Recap on Hope, Love, Fun—and Preparation

#146 *Constantly Innovate*

**Embrace Innovation:
Dating Demands Constant Growth**

Constant innovation is key to staying ahead in any field, and dating is no exception. Just like in business, where stagnation can lead to failure, a static approach in dating won't get you the results you're looking for. Simply posting a few photos and a short profile online and then waiting for things to happen is a surefire way to end up frustrated and blaming the process.

Adapt, Experiment, and Succeed

To succeed in dating, you need to be dynamic, constantly tweaking and improving your approach. If you're not getting responses to your messages, don't just sit back and wait—try something new. Maybe the messages you're sending are too generic; experiment with something quirky or unexpected. If your photos aren't attracting attention, switch them up. If your profile is too long or poorly formatted, streamline it into something more readable and engaging.

One client of mine, 63-year-old Becky, had what she believed was a fail-safe system and the "perfect profile", but it wasn't yielding the right results, eventually leading her to call me. By constantly innovating and adjusting Becky's approach—new photos, new prompts—she eventually found success. The lesson? In dating, as in business, you need to be willing to adapt, experiment, and continually refine your strategy. The key is to keep moving forward and not get stuck in one approach.

#147 Reminder: Get Out of Your Closed Mind Ways

The Power of an Open Mind: Lessons from Leadership and Dating

Having an open mind is crucial when navigating the dating world, much like in leadership, where good leaders are open to feedback. If you're not getting the results you want—like no one messaging you back—it's a clear sign that you need to change your approach and think outside the box.

I often compare online dating to a Target parking lot. When you go shopping at Target, you see all sorts of cars—BMWs, beat-up Toyota Corollas, Lamborghinis, Tesla's, and trucks. There's a mix of everything, just like you'll find on broad-based dating sites like Tinder, Bumble, Hinge, and Match. These platforms are full of diverse people from different walks of life.

Recap on Hope, Love, Fun—and Preparation

**Mastering the Filters:
Don't Settle for the First Swipe**

The key is to understand how to work the filters and algorithms to narrow down your search. Don't be discouraged by the initial likes or messages you receive; they often won't be the people you end up with. Instead, focus on actively searching and filtering for the type of person you're looking for. Having an open mind and staying proactive will help you navigate through the variety and find the right match.

#148 Seek Out A Mentor

In the business sector, mentors play a paramount role in guiding professionals through challenges and helping them achieve their goals. Nearly every successful business person has had a mentor who offered invaluable advice and perspective. The *Wall Street Journal* often highlights business leaders and their four mentors, who typically come from diverse backgrounds, bringing a wealth of experience and insight to the table.

Attributes of a Trusted Mentor

The same concept applies in the dating world. A healthy mentor in dating is someone who provides objective, constructive advice and helps you navigate the often-complex landscape of relationships. Here's how different types of mentors can benefit your dating journey:

1. The Experienced Friend: This mentor has been through the dating scene and understands the nuances of modern relationships. They offer practical advice based on their experiences, helping you avoid common pitfalls and encouraging you to stay optimistic.

2. The Objective Outsider: Sometimes, it's helpful to have a mentor who isn't directly involved in your social circle. This person can provide an unbiased perspective on your dating choices, helping you see things clearly and make informed decisions without emotional entanglement.

3. The Relationship Expert: Whether it's a therapist, coach, or counselor, a professional mentor can offer insights into your dating patterns, helping you break unproductive habits and develop healthier approaches to relationships. They can also equip you with tools to better understand yourself and what you genuinely want in a partner.

4. The Cheerleader: This mentor is all about boosting your confidence and reminding you of your worth. They encourage you to keep going, even when things aren't going as planned. Their positive energy can be infectious, helping you stay motivated and focused on your goals.

Recap on Hope, Love, Fun—and Preparation

5. The Tough Love Mentor: Sometimes you need someone who isn't afraid to call you out on your mistakes or challenge your thinking. This mentor provides the tough love that pushes you out of your comfort zone and helps you grow, both personally and in your dating life.

Each of these mentors brings something unique to the table, offering a balanced and comprehensive support system in your dating sojourn. Just as in business, having a diverse set of mentors ensures that you receive well-rounded advice, helping you to navigate dating with confidence and clarity.

#149 Pursue Professional Help When Needed

Prioritize Mental Wellness: Start with Professional Support

Navigating the emotional challenges of newfound singledom can be tough, especially if you're dealing with depression or inertia. Seek professional help when needed, and a good place to start is with your General Practitioner (GP). They can offer referrals to qualified therapists and, if necessary, help you find a psychiatrist for medication. Mental health is foundational—before diving into the dating universe, make sure you're feeling like your best self, or at least on the path to recovery.

The Importance of Healing First

If you're not feeling up to par, it's wise to pause and wait before jumping into the dating scene. Take the time to heal and regain your confidence. The journey toward mental wellness is just as important as the search for love.

#150 Hire A Dating Coach: A Strategic Investment

If you feel overwhelmed by the dating process or just need some guidance, a reminder here that hiring a dating coach might be the perfect solution. Choosing the right coach requires careful consideration:

Choosing the Right Coach

1. Speak on the Phone First: Ensure you've had a phone conversation with the coach before signing up. This will help you gauge if you're a good fit and if their style aligns with your needs. You'll be spending a lot of time interacting with this person, so you must like and trust them.

Recap on Hope, Love, Fun—and Preparation

2. Know Exactly What You're Paying For: Be clear on what the program includes. Some coaches offer vague promises without specifying what you'll actually receive. Make sure the services are spelled out—how much time you'll get, what specific activities they'll assist with, and how they'll support you throughout the process.

3. Choose Someone with 15-20 Years of Experience: Experience matters. A coach with at least 15-20 years in the business knows the dating landscape well. They've witnessed the evolution of dating markets and sites, and their longevity in the industry speaks to their legitimacy and effectiveness. These seasoned professionals not only rely on their own experience but often back it up with rigorous research, staying informed about trends and demographic shifts.

For instance, an experienced coach might have access to specialized data from sources like Pew Research or Gallup, which can provide insights into which dating platforms are thriving in your area. This level of expertise can make a significant difference in your dating journey, helping you target the right apps and strategies for your specific needs.

A dating coach isn't just a guide—they should also be your cheerleader and accountability partner. It's easy to feel discouraged and want to give up after a few weeks, but a coach will keep you on track, encouraging you to stay committed for the recommended three months.

Andrea McGinty

A good dating coach will be objective, not emotional. That's exactly what we need when dating.

Clients often find this accountability invaluable. Knowing that someone is watching, supporting, and holding them to their goals can be the push they need to keep going. Whether it's messaging a certain number of potential matches or refining your online profile, having someone there to check in with makes a world of difference.

For example, one client might call and say, "Did you see what I did online yesterday?" The coach, having kept an eye on their progress, can say, "Yes, I did. And I'm glad you did that because you knew we'd be talking today." This level of engagement keeps you motivated and ensures you're actively participating in the process, rather than just passively observing.

The combination of professional support, strategic advice, and consistent encouragement can transform your dating experience, making it not only more effective but also more enjoyable.

Recap on Hope, Love, Fun—and Preparation

#151 *Celebrate Successes— Even The Small Ones*

Celebrate the Little Wins: Fuel Your Motivation

In the dating vortex, just like in life, it is important to celebrate even the small successes. These moments keep you motivated and remind you that progress is happening, even if it's slow. I was fortunate to spend two days with Oprah and her crew, filming a couple on a date and later discussing it with Oprah on her show. We often think of Oprah as having the Midas touch, but her trek to mastery is a testament to the power of resilience.

Oprah Winfrey, an epitome of perseverance, faced numerous challenges before reaching her iconic status. Born into poverty, she was fired from her first job as a news anchor and made several failed investments, including a restaurant and a movie studio. Yet, she didn't give up. She kept going, learning from each setback, and eventually built a media empire.

Apply This Resilience to Your Dating Life

Adopt the same mindset to your dating game. It's easy to get discouraged, especially when things don't go as planned. Maybe you didn't get a response to your message, or the date didn't lead to a second one. Instead of focusing on what didn't happen, celebrate what did. Did you step out of your comfort zone and try a novel approach? Did you have a friendly conversation, even if it didn't lead to a relationship? These are victories, and they deserve recognition.

Just like Oprah didn't let her failures define her, you shouldn't let a few dating setbacks hold you back. Success in dating, as in business, often comes down to perseverance. Every small win brings you closer to finding the right person. Take a moment to celebrate those wins, no matter how small they may seem. They are all part of your journey toward success.

#152 Continuously Improve You

Stay Ahead:
The Innovation Mindset in Dating

The world's most successful companies—think Amazon, Intel, Samsung, Apple, and Coke—never stop improving. They understand that resting on their laurels leads to stagnation. They constantly innovate, adapt, and refine their strategies to stay ahead of the competition. The same principle applies to dating.

Recap on Hope, Love, Fun—and Preparation

Continuous Improvement: The Key to Dating Success

In today's fast-paced dating landscape, continuous improvement is key to staying competitive. How do you do this? By constantly updating your photos, revising your profile, and experimenting with different dating apps until you find the winning formula. If you're not getting the responses you want, it's time to change things up. Don't get stuck in a routine—keep evolving.

#153 Build High Self-Esteem

Confidence as Your Cornerstone

Believing in yourself is the foundation of successful dating. When you have confidence, like who you are, and take pride in what you do, you naturally attract others. High self-esteem allows you to present your best self, handle rejection with grace, and stay motivated even when things don't go as planned. Confidence is magnetic—when you feel good about yourself, others will too.

#154 Prioritize Self-Care

Avoiding Dating Burnout

Great leaders know that exhaustion and overwork can lead to disaster. The same goes for dating. Do you really want to go out on a date frazzled and exhausted? Prioritizing self-care is imperative. It's important to approach dating with a clear mind and a positive outlook, which means taking care of yourself first.

The Power of Self-Care

If you look at successful people, they often have routines that include relaxation, meditation, or even a simple practice like going to bed early. They know that a balanced life leads to better decision-making and a more positive presence—traits that are incredibly attractive in the dating field.

Recap on Hope, Love, Fun—and Preparation

#155 *Embrace Change*

Let Go of the "Old Days"

The dating arena, especially for those in certain age groups, doesn't work the way it used to. The sooner you embrace change and adopt a younger, more adaptable mindset, the happier and more successful you'll be. Plus, this mindset makes you more attractive to others. People are drawn to those who are open to new experiences and willing to evolve, rather than those stuck in their ways.

The Power of an Adaptable Mindset

I've said it before, and I will say it again: let go of the nostalgia for the "old days" when people met organically or "in the wild." Those days are gone, and it's time to adapt. By fostering a younger mindset, you'll not only navigate the modern dating landscape more effectively but also feel better about the process. Embracing change means recognizing that new methods can be just as successful, if not more so, than the old ways. This mindset shift will keep you open to new possibilities and opportunities.

Andrea McGinty

#156 Fake It 'til You Make It

Responding to Common Questions with Confidence

Some people shudder at this but get out of your own way because I see all the time… it works! Imagine you're out on a date, and they ask, "How's it going on Bumble for you?" The only answer you should give is, "Oh, so much fun! I've met some awesome people—just not the one yet." This is your response, even if you feel like bursting into tears or badmouthing the app.

Keep it positive. Projecting a confident and upbeat attitude will attract the right kind of energy and, eventually, the right kind of person.

The Joy of Success Stories

I truly love my clients. I mean, really, I do. Over the years, my career has introduced me to an incredibly diverse range of people—from Wall Streeters and ranchers to artists, engineers, doctors, and stay-at-home parents. I've met dog walkers, writers, politicians, tech enthusiasts, and gamers, to name just a few. The variety is endless, and I learn so much from every single one of them.

There's no better feeling than when I get that text, phone call, or photo saying, "Andrea, it worked!" That's when I feel like the happiest person on the planet.

Recap on Hope, Love, Fun—and Preparation

#157 People Aren't Always What They Seem

The Journey to Finding Love

Take Janie, a 62-year-old C-Suite executive from San Diego. She came to me wanting a long-term relationship, someone to grow with and travel. She'd never been married, had no children, and wondered about her "marketability." I reminded her it all depends on who she is and what she's looking for. Fun fact: many men who've been married before often prefer someone who's also been married and had children. When I asked Janie how she felt about dating a man who had kids, she said she'd love it. Her career had kept her from having children, but she was ready to embrace that in a partner.

On our first Zoom call, Janie was attractive but came across as distant, almost unfriendly. After two coaching calls and three dates, she was still cold, and even seemed frustrated with me. I was dreading our third call when, just before it, my teenage daughter overheard and said, "Mom, that lady is rude—just kick her out!" From the mouths of babes, right?

Andrea McGinty

A Happy Ending

But on that third call, something changed. Janie broke down in tears. Her mother had passed away just two weeks before she started working with me, and she had moved across the country to care for her. She was lonely and grieving. Suddenly, the cold exterior melted, and we finally connected.

Four months later, Janie met Adam. I spotted him because of his smile and his sailboat (she loves sailing!). This past Christmas, I received a card with pictures of the two of them, racing sailboats and traveling together. It was the best feeling ever.

- **Tip:** If you're a woman without kids but open to dating someone who has them, make it known in your profile! In Janie's profile, we made sure to say, "And if you have children, that's a huge plus for me—I'm the aunt who spoils her nieces and nephews." We turned what could have been seen as a "negative" into a strength.

Recap on Hope, Love, Fun—and Preparation

#158 Great Writers Don't Always Write Great Messages

A Quirky Misstep

Thomas, a 55-year-old widower from Washington, DC, is witty, goofy, and known for writing biographies. He came to me after five years of being single, ready to start dating again. I set him up with a killer profile and great photos and gave him his first homework assignment: write ten short messages to ten women, under three sentences each, and end with a question. Easy, right?

Well, on our next call, Thomas said he'd sent all ten messages but got zero responses. Puzzled, I asked him to forward me the messages. And there it was: instead of short, engaging messages, he was writing full-on novellas, complete with his quirky British humor—funny to those who knew him, but probably confusing to the women he was messaging.

The Turnaround

I rewrote a few messages for him, and four out of the five women responded. Three dates followed, and in July 2024, Thomas married one of them!

- **Tip:** Keep your messages short, sweet, and end with an intriguing question. Avoid generic lines like, "How's your Monday?"

ANDREA McGINTY

#159 Maybe Your Kids Know More Than You About Dating?

A Reluctant Start

Carli, 54, was a vibrant nurse who raised three daughters alone after being widowed. When her oldest daughter, Maria, heard me on a podcast, she gifted her mom a coaching membership with me for Mother's Day. Carli was less than excited, telling her daughters she didn't need to replace their father. But they wisely told her, "Mom, you're not replacing Dad, you're writing your next chapter."

Carli soon met Patrick, a 51-year-old widower with twin teen boys. They're now married, and Carli's daughters have embraced their new "little brothers" with open arms—though they lovingly refer to them as "beasts."

- **Tip:** You've still got a lot of life to live. Don't just live it for your kids or your career.

Recap on Hope, Love, Fun—and Preparation

#160 Sometimes, Mom Knows Best

A Mother's Determination

Lola, 87, called me out of the blue. She wanted my help—not for herself, but for her 51-year-old son, Todd. Described as a "nerdy, techy, gamer," Todd lived in Silicon Valley and had never been married. Lola purchased him a membership, though Todd was hesitant. During our initial Zoom call, Todd gave short answers while his best friend, Lisa, chimed in from the background, adding more details.

The Breakthrough

Lisa's insights helped me get to know Todd better, and together we found him the perfect match, Chrissy, a Google product manager. Lisa even served as Todd's "best woman" at the wedding. And Lola? She sent me a box of beautiful vintage clothes from her shop, which supplies costumes for movies. Every time I wear them, I think of Todd.

- **Tip:** Sometimes, moms and best friends know best!

Andrea McGinty

#161 It Might Not Be a Rebound After All

A Fresh Start after 20 Years

Alexa had been married to her college sweetheart for 20 years when they divorced at age 52. Just two months later, she attended the wedding of a couple I had set up and called me, eager to start dating. She was clear: no interest in marriage, just dating and having fun.

The Match That Changed Everything

Her second date with me was Mick, a high school history teacher. After their second date, Alexa called me and said, "I'm done with you, Andrea!" She'd fallen head over heels for Mick. Eleven years later, they're still happily married.

- **Tip:** Don't let others convince you it's "too soon" or that it's just a rebound. Follow your heart.

Recap on Hope, Love, Fun—and Preparation

#162 Your Type Might Not Be Your Type

Embracing the Unexpected

Kim, 63, came from the art world in NYC. She had only been married once, briefly, and her dates were always creatives. I suggested she step outside her usual type, and introduced her to Rick, an engineer from Westchester. Kim was hesitant but agreed to invite him to one of her gallery openings. Rick wasn't an artist, but he was curious about art and had a great sense of humor.

An Artistic Leap of Faith

Four years later, they're in a happy long-term relationship. They share wine dates and have proven that love doesn't always come in the package you expect.

- **Tip:** Don't be too rigid about your "type"—you might just be surprised!

ANDREA McGINTY

#163 Bonus Tips from Golden Bachelor Contestant

Finding love goes far beyond outward appearance. I know that may sound surprising in a world obsessed with marketing everything from foot creams to cosmetic enhancements but take a moment to look at the couples who stand the test of time. The women in those relationships aren't always 5'8" blonde Barbie dolls. They come in all shapes, sizes, and colors. Yet, they share certain qualities that keep their partners coming home.

The best part? You already have these qualities within you, waiting to be unlocked. With a little awareness and practice, you can rediscover the powerful, magnetic force of love that resides in you.

Here are ten beliefs and practices that my friend April Kirkwood (a contestant on 2023's hit show *The Golden Bachelor)* relies on when her magnetism dims:

Recap on Hope, Love, Fun—and Preparation

10 Beliefs and Practices by April KirKwood of *The Golden Bachelor*

1. Embrace your ageless soul. You are a soul that never ages. Laugh when you feel joy. Dance in your kitchen. Buy those go-go boots and strut! Let your inner child out to play, and watch your energy radiate like a breath of fresh air. Childlike wonder is contagious!

2. Harness your energy. You are pure energy—eternal, neither created nor destroyed. You have more power than you realize. Raise your frequency, and you will manifest the life you desire. Why stay tuned to AM when you can switch to PM and attract an equal vibration? Power is attractive!

3. Release guilt. You've done nothing wrong. You are a human, here to learn lessons about love. Romance can often feel like a test of your true purpose. When you're out in the world, silently send this message: *You are loved*.

4. Rituals for renewal. After every night comes the sunrise. When it does, practice three simple rituals: gratitude, affirmations, and setting intentions. These will help guide you through life's energy shifts, returning you to your best self.

5. Embrace solitude. There will be times you feel alone. This is a necessary phase of rest, reflection, and healing before new doors can open. Sometimes, the greatest inner growth happens when it looks like we're doing nothing. Pain is a teacher.

6. See relationships as assignments. Relationships are life assignments, each with a natural cycle. They are not failures or wastes of time. Ask yourself: *What was I meant to learn from this?*

7. Self-love precedes all love. You cannot truly love another until you love yourself, and they cannot love you until they've healed emotionally. If you choose to be with someone who doesn't understand your depth, know that they are like a child lost in the dark, searching for your light. You always have a choice.

8. Seek trust and safety. Most people are searching for someone they can trust and feel safe with. Remember, each person you meet is a reflection of God's light and deserves respect. Leave the games for the pickleball court and save the stoic face for meetings. Be real. Be you.

9. Don't take things personally. Don't be attached to outcomes. People often respond to only half of what's said, shaped by their own inner child issues. Stay positive and keep your energy aligned with peace—the highest frequency.

Recap on Hope, Love, Fun—and Preparation

10. Avoid these behaviors. Don't become obsessed with outcomes—it's off-putting. Don't fawn or play small—it creates the opposite of what you desire. Don't put anyone on a pedestal—when you do, you become the fan instead of the star of your own life. Remember, you are the lead in your own movie.

#164 Grit, Grit, and More Grit

Commit to Your Routine

Consistency is key to online dating success. Commit to a routine: for three months, spend 30-45 minutes, three times a week, engaging with your online dating profile. This isn't just a casual hobby—this is your love life. Think about the effort you put into hobbies like hiking or golf; now channel that same dedication into finding love. By maintaining a consistent presence, you increase your chances of making meaningful connections.

The Power of Commitment

Never give up on your quest for love. Persistence is key; the right person might be just around the corner. Even when the journey gets tough, keep going. Every setback is an opportunity to gain experience, grow, and get closer to finding the right partner. Perseverance is often the difference between success and failure.

Andrea McGinty

#165 Embrace The Waves of the Marketplace

Embrace Optimism on Your Dating Journey

Approach your dating adventure with optimism. Always expect the best possible outcome from your efforts. Your thoughts are powerful, like magnets—what you think, you attract. A positive attitude not only boosts your self-esteem but also makes you more attractive to others. Focus on the potential for success, and you'll be more likely to achieve it.

Stay focused on your goal and avoid the negativity of others. When Howard Schultz first talked about opening a coffee shop, people gave him strange looks, but that didn't stop him from creating Starbucks. In the same way, ignore the doubters, whether they're smug married friends or negative single girlfriends. Trust your instincts and stay true to your course.

Celebrate the Little Wins

Finding love is a journey, thus embrace every step of it. From the awkward first dates to the thrilling moments of connection, each experience contributes to your growth. Instead of focusing solely on the end goal, take time to appreciate the process. The ups and downs, the laughs, and even the missteps are all part of the adventure.

Recap on Hope, Love, Fun—and Preparation

Throughout your dating expedition, there will be plenty of moments that make you smile or laugh. Whether it's a funny text exchange or a sweet gesture on a date, these moments are worth celebrating. They remind you that the journey is just as important as the destination. Keep a sense of humor and cherish the heartwarming experiences along the way.

#166 Remind Yourself: You've Got This

Last But Not Least

As you enter the second act of your life, remember that love, life, and happiness are deeply intertwined. Finding love isn't just about being with someone; it's about enhancing your life and adding to your happiness. Embrace this new stage with an open heart and mind.

Be patient, stay positive, and know that your second act can be just as fulfilling, if not more so, than the first. I believe in you. I also believe in numbers. You've got this.

addendum
Worksheets #1-13

What you will find on the following pages are the worksheets I mentioned in the "How to Use This Book" section. These worksheets are fun, interactive, and easily printable.

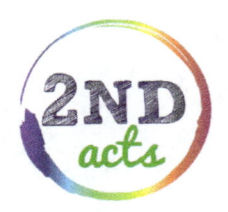

Worksheet #1: How to Rate a Dating Coach

What qualifies them as a dating expert?	
How long have they been coaching?	
Who are their typical clients?	
Is there a contact number?	
What are their fees?	
Do they revise profiles?	
Do they vet photos and suggest changes?	
Will they recommend suitable dating apps/sites?	
Do they assist with messaging?	
Do they provide feedback on initial dates and coach me on dates?	
How do they define success?	

33000Dates.com

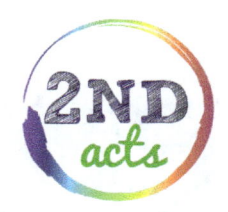

Worksheet #2: Am I Ready to Start Dating Again?

Am I feeling optimistic about dating?	
Do I feel like I can go on 1st and 3rd dates and not talk about my ex?	
Do I feel excited AND nervous about starting to date again?	
Am I professionally in a good place to have the time to devote to dating?	
Are my expectations reasonable? (List 3-5 non-negotiables.)	
Do I have a list of 10/20+ traits that are deal breakers? (Burn it.)	
Am I happy with my own life?	
Do I have friends and a sound support system?	
Am I active in my hobbies, sports, or passions?	
Do I have some confidence?*	
Am I committed to dating? (Not for the rest of my life but at least 2-3 months?)	

*Few people have 100% confidence going into dating, but we want you to believe you are a catch worthy of a fabulous partner!

33000Dates.com

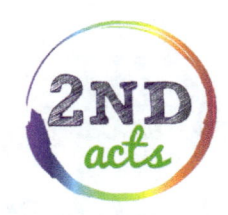

Worksheet #3: Personal Branding Brainstorm

Skills & Credentials	
Passions & Interests	
Values & Beliefs	
What do I want to be known for?	
What is my purpose and what am I trying to accomplish?	
What's the key message I want to convey?	
What personal traits do I want to showcase?	
What sets me apart from others?	
Who is my target audience?	
What feelings do I want my personal brand to inspire when someone sees me online for the first time?	

33000Dates.com

2ND acts

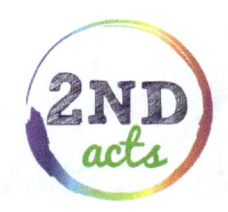

Worksheet #4: Plotting Your "Self-Reinvention"

What's my objective? (Do I JUST want to dip my toe into the dating waters or want marriage?)	
Text 3 friends and ask them for 5 adjectives to describe you that are not generic.	
What are my accomplishments? (Raising 3 kids? A stellar career? Awards?)	
Should I change my overall look?	
What don't I like about my life right now?	
What do I do for self-care?	
What do my 3 closest and most positive friends think I should change about myself before I start dating?	

33000Dates.com

Worksheet #5: Your Elevator Speech*

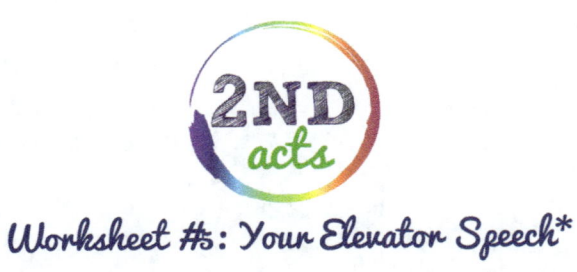

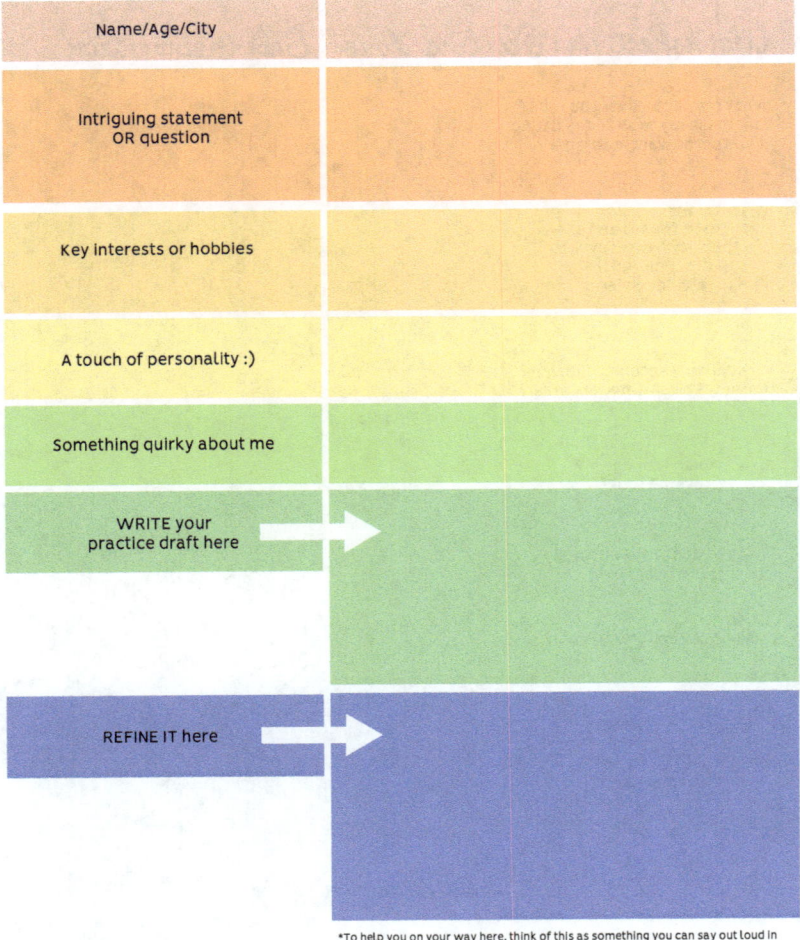

Name/Age/City	
Intriguing statement OR question	
Key interests or hobbies	
A touch of personality :)	
Something quirky about me	
WRITE your practice draft here →	
REFINE IT here →	

*To help you on your way here, think of this as something you can say out loud in 60-90 seconds max! No longer... short and sweet... or spicy!

33000Dates.com

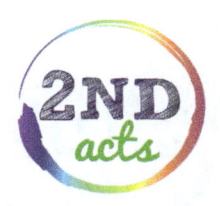

Worksheet #6: My Message Log

#	DATE	MESSAGES SENT	REPLIES BACK	PHONE CALL	DATE SCHEDULED
1					
2					
3					
4					
5					
6					
7					
8					
9					
10					
11					
12					
13					
14					
15					
16					
17					
18					
18					
20					
21					
22					

2ND acts

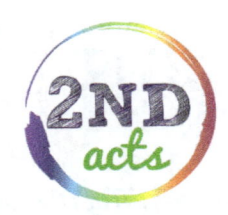

Worksheet #7: General Photo Checklist (a)

Do I have 4 different outfits?	YES ☐ NO ☐
Do I have props? (golf club, pickleball racket, book, dog, etc.)	YES ☐ NO ☐
What unique shots will I take outside?	
Do I have a shot of me sitting at a café with a coffee or glass of wine?	YES ☐ NO ☐
Where will I take my full body shots? (Don't just stand there—have a great background!)	
Can I take a sport shot? (on tennis court, hiking, lotus shot on a yoga mat, etc.)	
Can I take unique indoor shots at my home? (cooking, baking, reading in your library)	YES ☐ NO ☐
Have I changed my clothes at least four times? (1)	YES ☐ NO ☐
Do my teeth look great? (2)	YES ☐ NO ☐
Did I take at least one fun shot or bit of a goofy? (3)	YES ☐ NO ☐

33000Dates.com

(1) A client had great professional photos, but he wore the same outfit in all of them, so we could only use two. Gentlemen, just 4 different shirts with khakis or jeans can add variety!"

(2) My male client got tons of comments for his unique shot juggling pomegranates in a suit! (No need to juggle, but we're aiming for a memorable shot of you!

(3) Plan a week ahead: either book an hour at a medi-spa for great results or use Crest Strips daily for 7 days before the shoot.

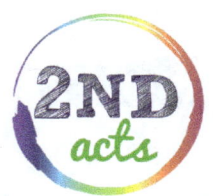

Worksheet #7: General Photo Checklist (b)

Checklist: For Men

Question	Yes	No
Do I look well-groomed, shaved, etc.?	☐	☐
Did I leave my baseball hat at home?	☐	☐
Did I take my glasses off for at least 2 photos?	☐	☐
Did I smile so viewers can see my teeth?	☐	☐
Did you get a recent hair cut?	☐	☐

Checklist: For Women

Question	Yes	No
Does my hair look great? (Hint: professional blow out)	☐	☐
Does my makeup look like me? (not overdone)	☐	☐
Do my nails look taken care of?	☐	☐
When I changed my outfits, did I change my earrings and necklaces?	☐	☐
When I wore lipstick, did I double apply it? (Yes, the camera needs this)	☐	☐
Did I take my glasses off for a few shots?	☐	☐
Am I comfortable in the clothes I chose?	☐	☐

33000Dates.com

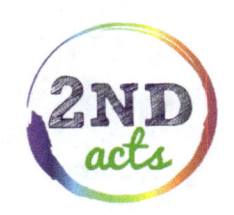

Worksheet #8: Am I a Positive Person?

What am I most grateful for?	
What am I most looking forward to or excited about?	
What am I most proud of?	
What makes me smile or laugh?	
Thinking of my closest friends, are they generally positive? What would they say about me?	
Do I make time for an active social life?	
Do I see mostly good in people?	
What are my top five positive traits?	
When I think of myself, do I mostly see my short-comings or strengths?	
Are most of my daily thoughts happy…or negative?	

33000Dates.com

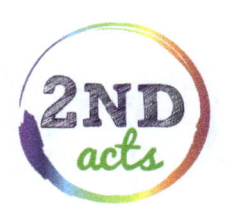

Worksheet #5: My Favorite Motivational Life Quotes

I'm going to start you off, then it's all yours!!

"When the going gets tough, the tough get going."
Attributed to both JFK and KNUTE ROCKNE

"If you don't like something, change it.
If you can't change it, change your attitude."
MAYA ANGELOU

33000Dates.com

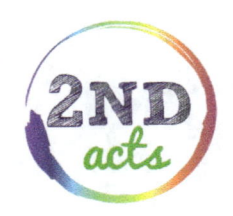

Worksheet #10: My Attitude Questionaire

Am I generally positive?	YES ☐	NO ☐
Am I open about others—cultures, religions, beliefs?	YES ☐	NO ☐
Am I happy with my life?	YES ☐	NO ☐
Do I have a good circle of friends who support me?	YES ☐	NO ☐
Do I laugh or exercise often?	YES ☐	NO ☐
Have I tried anything new this year, or have I made a new friend?	YES ☐	NO ☐
Do I get outside occasionally or eat somewhat mindfully?	YES ☐	NO ☐
Do I talk to "distance" friends occasionally? (yep, talk... not text)	YES ☐	NO ☐
Do I have a hobby I love and frequently engage in?	YES ☐	NO ☐
Am I curious, or do I read?	YES ☐	NO ☐

33000Dates.com

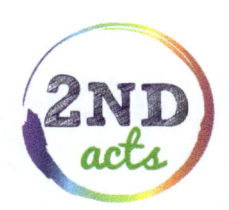

Worksheet #11: My One-Page Dating Plan

PROBLEM
What problem am I solving?

TARGET MARKET
Who is my target market?

COMPETITORS
Who are my competitors?

MARKETING PLAN
What is my marketing plan?

IMPLEMENTATION TIMELINE
What is my implementation timeline?

TIMELINE GOAL
What is my timeline to reach my goal?

PARTNERS
Is anyone else involved in my endeavor?

FUNDING
What funding is required?

33000Dates.com

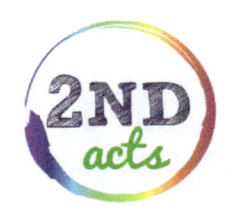

Worksheet #12: What Are My Dating Goals?

My dating goals for the next three months are...	
My ultimate goal is...	
I'm willing to do the following to achieve my goals Do I see mostly good in people?	
Why do I want to start dating now?	
Do I have any non-starters or obstacles?	
Do I want to find someone, or am I just lonely?	

33000Dates.com

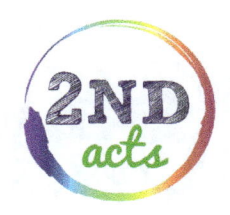

Worksheet #13: Putting my Profile Together for Online Dating Apps and Online Sites (a)

NOTE: You have done the work---hurray! Look back over Worksheets 3, 4, 5, 11 and 12 to save yourself time... and let's get rocking and rolling. Specific, interesting descriptions get attention. No time for generics, here, my friends!

What unique descriptions did my friends write about me?	
Do I have any "musts" such as religion, ethnicity, education, etc?	
What 3 things am I excited about that I do in my free time? (Be specific.)	
What is my profession?	
What makes me quirky? (Quirky is not weird! This could be a fun story or something you collect)	

33000Dates.com

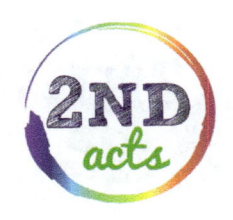

Worksheet #13: Putting my Profile Together for Online Dating Apps and Online Sites (b)

What are my favorite foods? (Be specific and descriptive as most people like to eat---and pasta is not an answer!)	
What makes me happy?	
What's the first thing my date will notice about me?	
What are my bucket list items?	
What 3 characteristics am I looking for in a date/LTR?	

33000Dates.com

Acknowledgments

In this book, I mention the importance of surrounding yourself with people you respect—who bring positivity and are experts in their field. I feel like I hit the lottery in that regard.

To HOLLIE MCKAY, my editor and friend—you are incredible. Working with you was pure joy, often accompanied by the sweet sound of little Raven baby-talking in the background. Your consummate professionalism and insights were spot on, and I'm still in utter shock that you took on my project. I admire your books and daily updates on current events—I don't know how you do it all! Although we're a generation apart, you completely understood the experiences of people over 50 reentering the dating world, and I learned so much from you. Bottom line: this book wouldn't exist without you.

To MICHAEL KLAUSNER—one of the most brilliant businessmen I've ever met. You've been bugging me for two years to write this book, and your thoughts, ideas, and inspiration finally kicked me in the butt and got this done! There's never been a conversation with you where I haven't walked away without two or three unique, solid ideas—thank you! You constantly challenged me, told me when things would or would not work, and never was a "yes man." And you always called a spade a spade, which I appreciated! I so much appreciate you always making time for me.

To my publisher, ROBBIE GRAYSON—who knocks me out daily with his ideas and sharp knowledge of this industry. His innovative recommendations and suggestions propelled this near-and-dear-to-my-heart project to completion. He accelerated my knowledge quickly from Publishing for Dummies 101 to an expert level, with perceptions and concepts unknown to me. You have taught me so much, Robbie, in a short time, and I'm grateful to Hollie for introducing us.

To KAT FLEISHMAN, my brilliant public relations mentor—for introducing me to so many people who helped with this endeavor. Even with you in Italy, you always made time for me, no matter the time of day. You are a marketing genius, not to mention a terrific writer in your own right. I am always overflowing with thoughts and smiling at the end of every Zoom call.

To my friend, APRIL KIRKWOOD—a contestant from Season 1 of the Golden Bachelor. Your contribution to my book was just lovely! The way you think about dating is thoughtful and on point. It's no wonder your vivacious, funny, and sweet self made it to this show, not to mention your success as an accomplished writer and speaker. I think the world of you!

And to my husband, JEFF QUINLAN—you are intelligent, analytical, and patient. Whether during a football game, on the golf course, or in the car, you were always open to my questions on men, dating, and the male perspective—no matter how obscure or awkward. You encouraged me throughout this writing process, and I can't thank you enough for keeping me balanced through it all. I said I'd never marry again, and here I am, in my "Second Act"—with the love of my life—thanks to online dating, no less! I'm so grateful you responded to my message and that our first date was on your birthday. Lucky me. I love you more every day.